A Primer for the Clinician Educator

This concise, introductory primer has been written specifically for clinician educators (CEs), particularly those new to the role and those working to further develop their experience and knowledge. Drawing on his dual roles as a pediatrician and medical educationalist, the author uses storytelling and personal experience alongside practical suggestions to support the reader in their teaching, patient care, and educational scholarship, helping both junior faculty and more senior educators to avoid pitfalls in all segments of their careers.

Key Features:

- Is accessible and informative for those new to teaching and more experienced clinician educators seeking to lead change
- Includes 35 top tips they don't teach in medical school or residency training
- Addresses key personal questions, such as "how do I approach my interview?", "how can I negotiate salary and benefits?", "how can I ensure a healthy balance between career and family life?", "how do I approach retirement?" and many more
- Is illustrated throughout with experiences from the author's distinguished career as a clinician and a pioneering educator

About the Author:
Larrie Greenberg, MD, is Professor Emeritus, Pediatrics, the George Washington University School of Medicine and Health Sciences, Children's National Medical Center, Maryland, USA.

A Primer for the Clinician Educator

Supporting Excellence and Promoting Change Through Storytelling

Larrie Greenberg

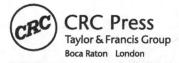

CRC Press
Taylor & Francis Group
Boca Raton   London

CRC Press is an imprint of the
Taylor & Francis Group, an **informa** business

First edition published 2023
by CRC Press
4 Park Square, Milton Park, Abingdon, Oxon, OX14 4RN

and by CRC Press
6000 Broken Sound Parkway NW, Suite 300, Boca Raton, FL 33487–2742

© 2023 Larrie Greenberg

CRC Press is an imprint of Informa UK Limited

The right of Larrie Greenberg to be identified as author of this work has been asserted in accordance with sections 77 and 78 of the Copyright, Designs and Patents Act 1988.

British Library Cataloguing-in-Publication Data
A catalogue record for this book is available from the British Library

Library of Congress Cataloging-in-Publication Data
A catalogue record for this book is available from the Library of Congress

ISBN: 978-1-032-28317-3 (hbk)
ISBN: 978-1-032-28316-6 (pbk)
ISBN: 978-1-003-29627-0 (ebk)

DOI: 10.1201/9781003296270

Typeset in Minion
by Apex CoVantage, LLC

Dedication

I am writing this primer for all the hardworking junior and mid-level clinician educators (CEs) who assume the majority of the responsibilities for patient care, teaching, and educational scholarship in our academic health centers. I am including some thoughts for the senior CE on three issues: retirement, as I feel this is a neglected area and not addressed by the academic health center, facilitation of workshops, and development of curricula with the contingencies that they teach others these skills, measure what they do, and publish these innovations with their junior colleagues, whether they be faculty or trainees.

This primer is dedicated to my supportive and loving wife, Joyce, of 57 years; my two wonderful children and their spouses (my daughter, Abby, and her husband, Shawn; my pediatrician son, Jeff, and his wife, Stefanie), all of whom have been caring and have flourished in their own rights; and my six grandchildren (Josh, Bradley, Jeremy, Adam, Jake, and Allie), with whom I have been blessed to have spent lots of time. Throughout my career, Joyce often asked me what I was doing when she saw me working on the computer. My answer, 95% of the time, was that I was editing some paper or writing something about education. I spent so many of my at-home hours doing this that I feel I owe her for taking time away from our relationship. She has been very supportive over the years.

I also owe sincere thanks to those who have mentored me over the many years spanning my career: E. V. Turner, MD (deceased), Columbus Children's Hospital (now Nationwide Children's Hospital); Richard Foley, PhD (deceased), the Center for Educational Development at the University of Illinois; Fredric Burg, MD (deceased), the University of Alabama School of Medicine; and Leslie Jewett, EdD, a colleague who was a vital part of the Office of Medical Education at Children's National Medical Center and collaborated with me on some of my initial educational scholarship. I also have valued my 25-year collaboration with Jim Blatt, MD, at The George Washington University School of Medicine, where we produced exciting and innovative programs and educational scholarship around teaching and learning.

Lastly, I dedicate this book to two of my wonderful friends and colleagues, Drs. Rich Sarkin and Steve Miller, superb clinician educators who were unbelievable models for the next generation of educators and whose lives ended way too early in a plane crash in 2004.

Contents

Preface

Before you start your journey through this book, I thought it would be helpful to address why an 81-year-old retired clinician educator (CE) would be writing a primer such as this. I have been busy finishing studies I began when I was working and was not necessarily looking for new ventures during this heinous pandemic. I did, however, have an epiphany as I was reflecting on some of my rich professional experiences and wondered if my personal stories wouldn't be helpful to those following in my footsteps.

In fact, a detailed online handbook by Turner et al.—*The Clinician-Educator's Handbook*—already exists, and my approach is not to duplicate that effort but to complement it, expounding on issues that those authors did not address through storytelling based on my personal experiences. In addition to the handbook mentioned earlier, a PubMed search revealed a few commentaries on how to be successful as a CE, but in my opinion, those articles lacked details and missed some key points that lead to excellence in academic medicine. Again, many of these missing points are illustrated in stories that have been an integral part of my career and my successes. It is not my intent to provide references on all that I write. In some places, where applicable, I have mentioned authors and articles throughout the book, and readers can easily Google them or go to PubMed or other search engines to access them.

I may have been one of the first, if not the first, CE focusing on education in pediatrics, and it is possible that some of my experiences might not be applicable to faculty today. In fact, I want to state up front that education has come a long way since I started my career. I am happy to say that those of us who made education an integral part of our careers in the 1970s and beyond were successful in our handoff to succeeding generations. When one looks at the spectrum of medicine today from 3,000 feet and sees what CEs are doing, many of them are leading the way in education. That was not the case when I started my career, when few faculty engaged in medical education as a major focus of their careers, and certainly, few role models encouraged this path. In fact, before physicians decided to make education a focus of their careers, nonphysician educators led the way and modeled for those of us primarily doing the work of CEs. Much of my early learning about the principles and application of education and educational scholarship was modeled by these PhDs involved in medical student and resident education. They laid the foundation for CEs. The value-added piece that has changed how we teach and learn is the ongoing information and technology explosion. Academic medicine is a different world today than it was just two decades ago.

I wanted to say a word about some of the publications that encouraged me to pursue writing this primer. Two books stimulated my interest in this publication: *Harvey Penick's Little Red Book: Lessons and Teaching from a Lifetime in Golf* by Harvey Penick and Bud Shrake, and *In Search of Excellence* by Tom Peters and Robert H. Waterman Jr. The two books feature stories from personal experiences and documented data, and contain either no references or only a handful of references. Both focus on ways to achieve excellence. The chapters are not necessarily sequenced, and the reader can choose a specific chapter to explore without having read information from the previous chapters. The authors tell lots of stories the reader can relate to, with lessons learned. I follow that model in this handbook, with the reader able to choose a specific topic without reading the book cover to cover. In each area of focus, I present stories that should resonate with the reader and lessons learned that can be carried forward as part of the change process.

Both *Little Red Book* and *In Search of Excellence* incorporate a theme of change. This theme is important in medicine—for getting patients to both adopt healthy lifestyles and change behaviors that are deleterious to their health, like obesity and smoking. The same adage applies to medical education, as the CE needs to be a messenger to induce change in teaching and learning based on evidence. As academicians, we have inherited traditions in teaching and learning, many of which are not evidence based. I emphasize the change process throughout this primer as it relates to the educational process, which applies across disciplines.

I was also encouraged to write this primer based on my 45 years of rich experience as a CE in pediatrics, with education being the focus of my career. So many stories have arisen over time that provide some lessons learned that will enable physicians to attain excellence with fewer roadblocks than I encountered. Rita Charon originated and popularized storytelling or narratives in medicine as a way to get trainees and faculty thinking about the humanities in medicine, and her work has been a nidus for every medical school in the US to incorporate humanities into the curriculum. Stories often tell so much about the persons involved—about character, work ethic, professional identity, ethical ideology, and interpersonal relationships, among others. The intent of using these anecdotes is to promote change using narratives that reflected my search for excellence as a CE, allowing the readers to assess the teaching points through their lenses.

Foreword

What clinician interested in medical education wouldn't treasure the chance for a series of fireside chats with a pioneer clinician educator? It is all here awaiting you. Larrie Greenberg, MD, is your host and mentor. In this book, he creates a casual, fireside setting and shares with you instructive and often poignant stories of his journey as a clinician educator, showing you the ropes in a way that can directly benefit your own career.

Dr. Greenberg is a general pediatrician, professor emeritus at the Children's National Medical Center, and former educational consultant to the George Washington University School of Medicine who has built his academic career around medical education. Dr. Greenberg dedicated himself to education as a career path in the late 1970s after special training from the Center for Educational Development, University of Illinois. There, he studied under such giants of the education world as George Miller, MD, Founding Director, Center for Educational Development, University of Illinois, Chicago. In 1979, Dr. Greenberg founded the Office of Medical Education at Children's National Medical Center, which houses the pediatrics department of the George Washington University School of Medicine. There, he became the center's leader in medical education and introduced learner-centered practices across the continuum, at the UGME, GME, and CME levels. Later, as educational consultant to the George Washington University School of Medicine, he (along with Rusty Kallenberg, MD, and myself) created and implemented Teaching and Learning Knowledge and Skills (TALKS): one of the first—if not the first—continuous formal students-as-educators programs in the country.

Dr. Greenberg's influence as a teacher and educator quickly moved beyond George Washington to the Northeast Group on Educational Affairs (NEGEA), where he rose to become chair of the steering committee. As chair, he strengthened the NEGEA by reaching out to schools that had been inactive and, through his contagious enthusiasm, energy, and personal commitment to the NEGEA, persuaded them to become actively involved. He was and is hard to resist. Dr. Greenberg's influence was also strongly felt nationally and internationally. He founded the Council on Medical Student Education in Pediatrics (COMSEP) in 1992 and became its president in the late 1990s. He has also served, by invitation, as a visiting professor in schools across the United States and in many medical schools in other nations.

Dr. Greenberg is what I can only describe as a *super-mentor*. I have seen him guide innumerable students, residents, and faculty in developing scholarship that resulted in countless presentations at national conferences and many, many publications. He does it by generously sharing his time and wisdom, by inspiring his protégés with his limitless energy and good spirits, and by bird-dogging them until they get the job done. I know all this firsthand: he has mentored me and innumerable others. When a colleague and I were asked about a mentor who was important to us personally in our careers, we both immediately cited Larrie as an exemplar—he has been a truly inspiration figure for each of us. Supporting our opinions are his many awards: he is a winner of the Miller-Sarkin Award from the American Pediatric Association as outstanding mentor in the country, winner of the Ray Helfer Award APA three times for outstanding research paper, winner of the George Washington University Distinguished Teaching Award, and recipient of a special recognition by GWU (the George Washington Award) and University of Toledo for lifelong contributions in education.

Dr. Greenberg is not only a super-mentor; he is one of the most prolific clinician educator scholars in the field of medical education. He has over 300 national presentations and more than 250 peer-reviewed medical education publications to his credit. He was the first to do a randomized controlled trial to assess a residents-as-teachers program and broke new ground by using standardized patients to study residents' communication skills with families in emergency situations.

Dr. Larrie Greenberg is a medical education pioneer, a Johnny Appleseed who sowed the joy of a medical education career in the hearts of so many young clinicians years ago, when the field was not well known among physicians. He is also a father of NEGEA, deeply committed to it and its mission, moving it forward as a member and, ultimately, as its chair.

In this book, Dr. Greenberg continues his mentorship, extending it to a fortunate larger public. He has organized it into chapters addressing the early, middle, and late phases of the clinician educator career.

Covering the entire spectrum of the clinician educator's professional life, each chapter is divided into the following sections: teaching, patient care, educational scholarship, advocacy, mentoring, and administrative responsibilities and leadership. The cherry on top is a series of 35 tips, many of which could vitally impact a career. So settle in and prepare yourself for some great storytelling. In Larrie's own words, "Knowing that you have effected change perhaps forever in a positive way that will make patient care better is as good as it gets! It answers the statement 'I know when I am teaching . . . I need to know if you are learning.' When you see it in-vivo with your very eyes, it's magic." This is your opportunity to share in the magic and be inspired to create some of your own.

Benjamin Blatt
Professor of Medicine and Medical Director,
CLASS Clinical Skills Center
The George Washington University School of
Medicine and Health Sciences
Washington, DC

Author Biography

Larrie Greenberg was born in Toledo, Ohio, in 1940, graduating from the University of Toledo with a BS degree in 1961 and graduating from medical school at the Ohio State University School of Medicine in 1965. He completed his pediatric internship at Buffalo Children's Hospital in 1965–1966 and returned to Columbus Children's Hospital where he completed his pediatric residency and chief residency in 1969. He served two years in the Army at Kimbrough Army Hospital from 1969 to 1971 and then was the pediatrician at Alyn Orthopedic Hospital in Jerusalem from 1971 to 1972. Upon his return to the US, he spent a year at Johns Hopkins before being recruited by Children's Hospital and The George Washington University School of Medicine and Health Sciences in 1974 to initiate a community hospital rotation for pediatric residents and medical students. In 1978, he created the Office of Medical Education at Children's National Medical Center. He has more than 300 publications, having published over seven decades; has greater than 340 national presentations; and has been a visiting professor in medical education at two-thirds of US medical schools. He has been the recipient of many awards for his educational scholarship, mentorship, curricular innovations, and lifetime achievement awards. He was likely one of the first, if not the first, pediatric clinician educator in the country, making education the focus of his career. His current passions include seeing his family and friends, staying connected to academia through ongoing studies and review papers, gardening, listening to jazz, traveling, exercising, and catching up on lost time with his wife, Joyce.

Introduction

1

As I am writing this handbook specifically for academic physicians who are clinician educators (CEs), the first order of business is to define that term. In essence, these are the physicians who assume the major responsibility for patient care, teaching, and educational scholarship in our academic institutions (Greenberg, *Acad Med.* 2018;93:1764–1766). Many are part of a community of learners, such as clerkship directors and residency program directors, where they convene at national meetings with a common interest in medical education and represent a large segment of those who have assumed leadership roles in medical education within their departments and medical schools. The majority of these faculty reside in general medicine (primary care), emergency medicine, intensive care medicine, and hospitalist divisions or departments. Some CEs may be subspecialists, surgeons, and a smattering of others who are responsible for specific areas, such as ethics and child protection. Whereas my perspective as a CE is from a physician point of view, there are many faculty in our academic health centers who are not physicians but are integral to providing interdisciplinary care to patients, including physician assistants, nurse practitioners, physical therapists, psychologists, dentists, pharmacists, and others. All these faculty devote much of their time and energy to patient care, and along with that, they assume the major teaching responsibility for training future healthcare professionals as part of their job description. They are generally not tenured, they are often on a clinician promotion track, and most of their research does not involve large grant funding. That is not to say that they do not do research, and I will address that when discussing educational scholarship. Their promotions along the academic ladder are generally on the basis of their teaching expertise and educational scholarship. This definition of CEs is in contrast to clinician scientists, who spend most of their time (at least 70%) focusing on research and devote limited time to patient care, teaching, and educational scholarship. Finally, pediatrics places a high value on advocacy as part of its academic mission. I address these issues pertaining to the CE in subsequent chapters.

In today's world, most specialties value education and are allotting more resources to make education work at the medical school and departmental levels. Lest we forget, education is not a revenue center and represents a cost to institutions. On the other hand, there are monetary pass-throughs from Medicare and Medicaid to specifically support resident education, and those who value education realize they have the responsibility of training and modeling for future physicians.

MY EARLY EXPERIENCES IN THE FIELD

My first academic job in 1972 was at a well-known East Coast institution where I served as an ambulatory physician and oversaw residents, medical students, and a new group of health professionals called nurse practitioners. Whereas the position had some wonderful aspects to it—namely, I had my own module of patients, receptionist, nurses, medical records, and trainees (medical students and residents)—I realized early on that the institution did not value primary care or its providers. After eight months or so, I began looking for another academic position and received a letter from the Children's National Medical Center in Washington, DC, asking if I would be interested in starting a pediatric program in a community hospital affiliation with Children's and The George Washington University School of Medicine and Health Sciences. The letter stated that I was an excellent candidate and was an outstanding teacher.

I assured my wife that I was going to interview for the position but surely would not accept any offer, as we were headed back to the program where I did my residency training, Nationwide Children's Hospital in Columbus, Ohio. My interviews were, for the most part, with practicing pediatricians affiliated with the hospital in Silver Spring, Maryland, as well as leadership from Children's Hospital and the medical school. Basically, the position was created for a pediatrician to start de novo a community hospital rotation for residents and medical students, a novel idea at a time when the concept of community medicine was evolving.

Retrospectively, it did not seem that anyone was interested in my educational credentials or how I would navigate establishing this community-based connection to academic institutions. Maybe they were stuck on my being ascribed an excellent teacher, but in the end, they offered me the job, starting in January 1974. I accepted the position, with the support of my spouse, and immediately started to focus on what I thought needed to be addressed in the community that was not happening in the academic centers.

Upon reflection, a number of issues and potential problems came to mind:

1. I had no experience as a trained educator, and here I was in charge of a major eight-week rotation for residents and a four-week rotation for medical students, their only community experience.

2. I had never written a curriculum before, which would have included goals, objectives, and evaluations of experiences at the resident and medical student levels.

3. I wasn't certain what the curricular content should be, vis-à-vis how it would fit with the overall curricula at Children's Hospital and George Washington University.

4. I had a major responsibility was to oversee the education and patient care on the inpatient and neonatal units. The role of the practicing pediatricians who were admitting children to this inpatient unit and were referred babies in the nursery was not specifically verbalized. It was clear to me that when questions about patient care arose and there were differences of opinion between the admitting physicians and the residents, I would likely be the arbiter.

5. I was concerned that teaching responsibilities also were unclear, including who would assume those, in addition to me.

6. I recognized early on that this affiliation evolved between Children's and GWU as an inpatient rotation and yet was supposed to provide a community experience in how practice works, not just involving inpatients. The question would be posed as to whether this was a representative picture of community practice and this disconnect would lead to an office rotation for residents as part of their community experience.

7. I realized that, for better or worse, the leadership at Children's had a hands-off approach to this rotation and, in essence, was gauging its success by resident and student feedback. My perception was that educational leaders at the mother institution were not focused on the theory and principles of education (not unusual for that genre) and that I was on my own, which in the long run was a blessing for me.

Lessons learned: When you are just starting a new position, there is so much to know and often very little advice coming from others around important issues. It's almost like each challenge can be a trial by fire experience (i.e., you can't really know it until you are immersed in it yourself). That was 100% true in my case, and there are positives and negatives for this model. The senior leadership at Children's really let me fly on my own and offered suggestions when I asked but did not proactively offer guidance. Even though I was a very junior faculty member, this approach allowed me to experiment, take chances, grow, and mature academically far faster than had I been closely mentored by someone with more experience. Since I essentially was given full reign of my responsibilities, the bottom line was that leadership was looking for a return on investment in the success of the program. I will address in a later section how current faculty who are invested CEs can be of major assistance when one is starting a new position as opposed to trial by fire.

Truth be told, there were few role models with any educational background either at Children's or the medical school in the '70s who could have been significant mentors to me, aside from perhaps developing a curriculum. My subsequent experiences visiting more than two-thirds of pediatric departments or medical schools throughout North America in the 1980s and 1990s suggested that the chairs of departments did not always value education, as evidenced by a lack of significant funding in this area, and few academic pediatricians had any educational backgrounds or interest in education in those days. Early on, family medicine departments seemed to lead the way in supporting CEs in educational efforts as opposed to those in internal medicine and pediatrics.

The other telltale evidence about the status of education in the academic community in the 1970s and early 1980s was that the scholarship that CEs produced was not often published in specialty journals. In my case specifically, many articles that I would have preferred to publish in pediatrics were published in educational journals, like *Academic Medicine* and *Medical Education*, which, parenthetically, were seldom read by my colleagues. In those days, specialty journals did not appear to have a cadre of reviewers who felt competent to assess educational studies and, more specifically, qualitative studies, and I am convinced that fellow physicians did not value that kind of research. Thus, the most likely place to publish educational scholarship was in medical education journals. Over time, that has changed, and specialty journals are now more open to educational scholarship.

Another short story will illustrate a point about the importance of educational expertise. When I was informed that I was considered an excellent teacher in my letter of recommendation for the community hospital position, I was flattered but not certain it was accurate. Not knowing some of the underlying theories of education, how would I have known about my teaching performance? So began my travails into faculty development. In those days, one could obtain a master's in medical education in a couple of places throughout the country, and occasional faculty development workshops were advertised, usually by family medicine faculty, that one could attend. I serendipitously happened upon a three-day workshop in Chicago that focused generally on teaching and learning. I was clueless in terms of what I needed to learn in medical education (in retrospect, everything) but thought this would be a good maiden voyage into the field.

My memory is not so clear, having been to that workshop 45 years ago, but I distinctly remembered learning that I was not a great teacher—but a great information-giver. In essence, that workshop and my responsibility as the sole full-time faculty person in this community hospital stimulated my further exploration of medical education. That three-day workshop provided me with a new language that I never imagined I could master, as my baseline educational knowledge was close to zero. It opened a whole new world for me and challenged the status quo with which I was so comfortable. I was inspired and stimulated to seek more of the same.

Another chance happening significantly impacted my career in the late '70s. As chance would have it, Richard Foley, PhD, a faculty member from the then Center for Educational Development at the University of Illinois (now the Department of Medical Education), consulted at George Washington University on lecturing skills, and I enthusiastically elected to participate in his workshops. It was intimidating to me to listen to the previously unknown theoretical constructs underlying the lecture and then apply that new knowledge by lecturing in front of peers. I received feedback and then had to use that feedback in redoing the lecture. Dr. Foley became my first mentor, and when I spoke with him over a number of occasions, he suggested that spending time at the Center for Educational Development would be beneficial for my career. Eventually, I spent an initial two weeks there, speaking with many faculty and reading basic educational books aimed at undergraduates studying to be teachers about curriculum, teaching, evaluation, and learning.

Probably the most impactful experience for me at the University of Illinois was meeting Dr. George Miller, an internist who is considered the father of medical education. At our meeting, when I related what my responsibilities were in the community hospital, he told me that it sounded interesting and then asked, "What are you doing to effect change?" I had no answer. He promptly got up from his chair and pulled a couple of books that pertained to change off his voluminous bookshelves. He stated that change was the essence of teaching (i.e., getting people to learn more effectively and apply that learning to patient care or education).

Lastly, in 2000, when I segued into a position later in my career that challenged me to develop a faculty development program on the main campus at George Washington, a faculty member in the School of Public Health who was very committed to educational excellence told me that he was in an elevator on his way to the office and overheard two surgeons speaking about my appointment. One said to the other, "What could a pediatrician possibly tell us about teaching and learning?" This is such an important learning point in that there is a misconception that education is more about content rather than process. The content expertise of the teacher should never be the focus of the change process—only how effectively the education is delivered to learners.

I doubt that my early experiences are typical of what happens in academic health centers today, but seeking out faculty with an interest in education is key when you start a new job. You are looking for allies with similar interests whom you can call on to offer suggestions and advice, and to converse with about educational issues. In most divisions or departments and medical schools, many faculty are invested in education, and making a point to seek out some of these people can be the beginning of enduring collaborations. You also will be thinking of how to show leadership the value of what you do educationally through your teaching and educational scholarship.

THEME: EFFECTING CHANGE

When starting a career as a CE, asking the question of how to effect change is quite an important one. Espousing evidence-based truths is not enough in engaging trainees and faculty in medical education activities. Engagement requires perspective-taking (i.e., putting yourself in someone's shoes to understand their perspective and directing your education to meet their needs). It also is showing passion in what you do and making each encounter seem as if it were the first. An example is having participants advise you on where they feel they need help, like dealing with the problem learner or observing trainees effectively. Developing evidence-based workshops that address these issues, using a hands-on approach and opportunities to practice newfound knowledge, is essential for promoting effective learning.

Promoting change is a principle integral to adult learning theory. I am guardedly optimistic that my personal stories will resonate with CEs and help them through the change process. The theme of change in medicine is so important for getting patients to adopt healthy lifestyles and change behaviors that are deleterious to their health, like obesity and smoking. The same adage applies to medical education, as the CE needs to be a messenger to induce change in teaching and learning based on evidence. As academicians, we have inherited traditions in teaching and learning, many of which are not evidence-based. I emphasize the change process throughout the primer as it relates to the educational process, which applies across disciplines.

THEME: INNOVATION AND COLLABORATION

The small but poignant book *Who Moved My Cheese: An Amazing Way to Deal with Change in Your Work and Your Life* by Johnson is very applicable to what we do every day in medicine. It discusses change in terms of growth and innovation. We don't grow academically unless we take chances and seek new ways to teach and effect learning that are fun and enduring.

We are not always successful in what we do—sometimes because we have not sought collaborators who can add value to our ideas about innovations and scholarly activities. We also come up short in evaluating what we do, leading to questions about the efficacy of an innovation. This being said, I loved taking risks and always saw myself as an idea man, realizing almost 100% of the time that I needed people on board who had expertise in methodology and statistical design. If you examined my CV (which makes for boring bedtime reading), you would see the scores of collaborators I have enlisted (or been enlisted by) in innovations and educational scholarship. I am still engaged in important projects that I am confident will reach closure at some point and be published.

THEME: SEEKING EXCELLENCE

The search for excellence has been a mantra for me since I started my academic career. I stated to myself (and sometimes out loud) over and over how I set my overall goal to make a difference in academic medicine. I really had no idea how that vision was to play out, but I continued to reflect on this goal in all that I did, trying to make myself better as well as the institution. I wasn't ever able to settle for less. I indeed strove to achieve excellence, always an ongoing battle.

ORGANIZATION OF THE BOOK

The four major components of excellence in education are the teacher, the learner, the curriculum, and the learning climate. Details on each of these components are provided elsewhere, as in Turner et al.'s *The*

Clinician-Educator Handbook, available online. This primer addresses those four components within the context of the CE's teaching responsibilities and enumerates tips for different levels of the CE's career.

The first three chapters address the CE career temporally (i.e., the early, mid, and late periods). Within the early and mid-levels of an academician's career, I address patient care, teaching, educational scholarship, and advocacy. For senior-level CEs, I address retirement decisions, their role in conducting evidence-based workshops that can be models for change, and hand-offs to the younger faculty.

I also include a chapter on tips based on poignant critical incidents in my career. For some, these tips might be old hat and not applicable to their current situation as CEs. For others, these tips might be vignettes that inspire and challenge them to think about what they are doing and how that can be reinforced and/or improved. Lastly, I include an annotated bibliography of ten books that had a significant influence on my knowledge and performance in education. These are meant to be representative and not all-inclusive, and some may be out of print. Educational principles and practice are tried and true over time and are seldom outdated. For example, when you read Knowles' work on andragogy, I am certain it will resonate with you as to your own knowledge and practice. So don't let the old publishing dates bias you.

The Chapter 2 begins with the junior clinician, commenting on obtaining that first position in the field and addressing its myriad responsibilities.

2

The Junior Clinician Educator

Since this chapter addresses the junior clinician educator (CE), a logical place to start is the hiring process and how novice faculty traverse that initial interaction with the academic institution. What I offer here are some insights regarding going through the interview process, negotiating a job description and salary, assessing what the job entails, and recognizing your need to be successful in your career. I then address different components of the role: patient care, teaching, educational scholarship, advocacy, mentoring, and administrative responsibilities.

OBTAINING AND NAVIGATING YOUR FIRST CE POSITION

I use the word *career* in this description rather than a *job*. For some who read this handbook, developing a career versus having a job is an important differentiation. I see a career as a longitudinal piece of one's professional identity and development that evolves over time and can morph into specific interests and paths, hopefully leading to excellence and success. On the other hand, there are those who want a connection to teaching, with their primary focus being patient care. They place high priority on family life versus professional advancement and likely view educational scholarship as an additional burden to their day. Individuals who choose this path might also not work full-time because of their family obligations.

DOI: 10.1201/9781003296270-2

Preparation for the Interview

Once a job interview is scheduled, what do you need to think about beforehand? Here are some issues I consider critical for the interviewee to know before the in-person or, in the case of the COVID-19 pandemic, the virtual interaction:

- What does the institution's website look like and what information is listed that would be helpful in your decision about wanting to work there? You also should be thinking about information that you feel is important that may *not* be part of the website. Being knowledgeable about what appears on the website may present talking points as you navigate the interview process. Speaking with colleagues in the business world and other disciplines can often be helpful regarding points to discuss and ask about during the interview.
- What is the specific job description and does it fit your mission statement? You might have questions about specific details and/or areas not mentioned for the division or department in which you will be working, like frequency of night call, supervisory responsibilities, specific teaching activities, maternity/paternity leave, vacation and sick leave time, keeping of an educator portfolio, and availability of mentors, to name a few. Specifically ask what the program expects from you as it pertains to the mission of the academic health center, that is, teaching, patient care, research (educational scholarship), and in some specialties, advocacy. Note that the days of being a triple threat are over, and the expectation to excel in all three to four areas of the academic mission is unrealistic. Just make certain you know what is expected from you so there are no hidden agendas and you can focus on an area in which you can excel.
- What resources are available for you in the program and at the medical school to increase your knowledge and performance in this area, if teaching is to be a major responsibility (which is often the raison d'être for choosing academic medicine)? Faculty development is important to the growth of junior CEs, and segueing into that mode early in your career will pay long-term dividends. Faculty development exposes you to innovative facilitators conducting workshops and to participants in those workshops with common educational goals, often enabling lifelong collaborations and friendships. I would suggest that your onboarding package include expenses paid for travel to a national educational program, like the Society for General Internal Medicine, the Academic Pediatric

Association, the Association of Surgical Educators, or more generally, the Association of American Medical Colleges.

- What are the salary, fringe benefits (health insurance, malpractice insurance, disability insurance, profit-sharing plan, and vacation and sick time), and academic appointment? Usually, the position is on a non-tenure track, and in many institutions, it is at a clinical level (i.e., clinical assistant professor). In some cultures and countries, salary depends on years of experience since completing medical school and is not negotiable. Having been in an administrative position, I can tell you the once the institution offers you a job, salary will usually be addressed, and in many instances, division or department heads are given a range for the position. When I was negotiating my position at Children's in 1973, I was offered a salary of $31,000. A friend in business suggested that I tell them that I was looking for a higher salary. I did that and received $34,000, a significant increase in those days. (Retrospectively, I probably could have asked for more but was hesitant and not confident to do so.) The downside is that one has to be very confident and able to retreat if the hiring manager indicates that the salary offered is the going rate for the position.

The Interview Process

For the interview process itself, the best advice I can give is to recognize that there are likely many other people vying for the same position. Here's an important question: Why should that program choose you? To answer that question, you have to come across as committed, passionate about what you do, and knowledgeable about the specific area in which you are applying and about the overall program. Having some specific interests in starting academic life can also be a good talking point. As an example, if you are applying for a position as a hospitalist, what do you know about the program and the current faculty in the program? Some of the current mid-level and senior faculty may have leadership positions in national organizations or be well-published in certain areas. You might distinguish yourself from other applicants by stating specifically that you feel there is an absolute fit between you and the program and explaining why. Your interests can also be in sync with the mission of the department. As an example, our ob-gyn department, with whom we worked extensively on developing a residents-as-teachers program, prides itself on being committed to teaching. If that is your passion, that would be a very nice fit. Also, don't be afraid to bring to the interviewers' attention awards you have won, how you have excelled (this could be from recommendations or evaluations you have received), and why offering you a position would be a win-win proposition for you and the program. Be humble when you advocate for yourself, but remember there are others being considered. I have found this approach to be rewarding in my career when competing against candidates who sometimes had better credentials.

Following the interview, send an email summarizing what you think transpired. Mention that you appreciate the opportunity and that your impressions about the program have been confirmed and have piqued your interest even more. Indicate that you look forward to hearing from them soon. It is reasonable to send another email a few weeks later to reconfirm your interest in the program and ask when they will decide on a candidate.

Beginning a Position

Following the interview process, you receive an email and a letter offering you the position. One of the first orders of business to prepare you for what lies ahead is to develop a mission statement, if you haven't done that already. How would you describe who you are professionally and what you want to accomplish academically? I would suggest that your mission statement be 30 words or less and provide a snapshot if someone asks about your vision and goals as a junior CE. This is a difficult exercise for even seasoned physicians, but it makes you focus on your passion and what you want to do to be successful at this point in your career. An example of a mission statement would be the following:

> My passion is to excel in patient care and teaching, and I want to do collaborative educational scholarship in the field of community health.

The other important point is to refer back to your mission statement when you are asked to take on new responsibilities. New ventures that are offered to you can be flattering and interesting, but it all comes back to what you are all about, as expressed in your mission statement. As an example, when someone asks you to be involved in immunization surveillance and this is not something that fits your mission statement, you would be able to say no without reservations.

As you start your new position, you will be completing tasks inherent in any new job, like surveying the physical plant where you will be working, getting introductions to colleagues, and meeting nonphysician healthcare workers who are a vital part of the team. As you acclimate to your new position, some important issues may arise in regard to your roles, responsibilities, and expectations.

As an example, you might observe, through notations in the medical record, that the diagnosis of otitis media is not being accurately described, and therefore, it would appear that patients older than two years are being inappropriately provided antibiotics based on inaccurate recordings of the diagnosis. As a junior staff member, going through channels seems to be the better part of valor, and in this case, letting the division chief know of your concern is appropriate. Perhaps this would morph into a continuing professional development educational session that you could lead and/or a quality improvement review for the division. Being careful not to point fingers at individuals but to address issues more generally and systemically could result in behavioral change and better care for patients. These kinds of critical incidents can be recorded in your educator portfolio, noting the intervention and the change that occurred. Repeated incidents like this can be great documentation when the time comes for promotion to the next academic level.

I had an experience that can illustrate how you can take advantage of situations when the job description is general and allows room for innovations. When I agreed to take my second academic job in a community hospital associated with Children's Hospital in Washington, DC, the overall goals were stated quite clearly, although many unforeseen gaps were not addressed that required some decision-making and negotiating along the way. One issue that arose that I had not thought about during my job interview was defining the resident experience in the community hospital. I maintained that an inpatient rotation was not representative of a community experience, and I proposed an office-based curriculum as an answer to that gap. When I approached the leadership at Children's about this, they advised me to negotiate with the chief executive officer at the community hospital. He was not happy about this, as the contract between Children's and this hospital called for paying the salaries of four residents to perform inpatient duties. I assured him that this office experience would enhance the quality of the rotation and that patient care would not be compromised by rotating residents through community offices over a two-week period. Ultimately, residents spent one week in a solo practitioner's office and one week in a group practice. The overall goal was to enlighten residents about practice in the community, with an emphasis on ambulatory care. The curriculum focused on topics, such as hiring and firing personnel, maintaining office records, dealing with referrals, providing telephone medicine, and billing. This office experience became a highlight of the rotation, providing residents with a look at the specialty from a practitioner point of view. The lesson learned here is that keeping open to what works and what needs to change as you navigate your new position is important.

PATIENT CARE

The most important area in terms of time involvement for every CE is patient care, and one of the challenges is how to measure your effectiveness and efficiency in providing this care. Most hospitals do exit surveys of patients and families in the ambulatory and inpatient settings to assess these issues, but the answers may not always be accurate for many reasons. One reason is patients' concern that their responses may not be totally anonymous; they might assume that being critical of the experience might affect their care in the future.

Better than patient exit surveys are quality improvement projects around patient care metrics. Since external and internal forces dictate how effective care is, you should determine what quality improvement projects are already in place that measure care so you don't reinvent the wheel. If there aren't any of interest, developing a quality improvement project for the team might be an option. If you measure outcomes in a rigorous manner, you can publish papers on quality improvement projects, and this can count as scholarship in building a curriculum vitae.

One example would be to place calls 24 hours after the visit to all patients who present with a sore throat, with one group testing positive for streptococcal pharyngitis and the other group having non-streptococcal pharyngitis. You could assess issues, such as continuance of symptoms, return to activity, patient-perceived importance of the call, and follow-up instructions (like taking antibiotics for the full treatment or returning to the ambulatory center if symptoms do not improve in 48 hours). The important point here is that if you consider patient care your main responsibility as a CE, it is incumbent upon you to measure how effective your care is through quality improvement studies that address patient safety, costs, effectiveness of care, outcomes, readmissions, timeliness of care, and mortality. Often, resources are available within the division or department that can provide important perspectives on a problem and even help with data collection.

Segueing into another aspect of patient care, it is important for the CE to teach skills and provide tips to trainees in performing the history and physical exam. In your journey as an academic physician, you will learn many nuances along the way that become valuable teaching points as a way to assess patients. I address these in the next section on teaching. In academic medicine, the lines are blurred between patient care and teaching (i.e., you can do patient care *and* teach trainees about some of the nuances you observe). The most effective teaching is performed at the chairside or bedside, where the teacher and the learner can see change evolve, within the context of patient care, right before their very eyes. This in vivo experience involves translating information learned in the classroom and applying it to the patient. Importantly, soliciting feedback from trainees about how you assisted them in providing patient care is paramount in building your educator portfolio.

Several stories illustrate how being astute and observant in doing a history and physical can be helpful to trainees. My favorite teaching moment is having trainees stand at the doorway of a room and observe the patient before interacting or examining him. I was on teaching rounds with a small group of third-year medical students on the pediatric clerkship, and we were visiting a patient unknown to them. Before entering the room, I asked the students what they saw, and surprisingly, they were not as observant as they could have been. The patient was a preadolescent with cystic fibrosis who was in bed, sitting in a forward position, with increased respirations. When we entered the room and approached the patient, the signs of obstructive pulmonary disease were more obvious to them. The learning point was self-evident: Before engaging the patient, observe the patient for signs of disease that will provide clues to the diagnosis.

I then tell them a famous story about William Osler, the most distinguished professor of medicine at McGill and Johns Hopkins in the late 19th and early 20th centuries. He took medical students to the bedside of a diabetic patient, suggesting that they observe the patient first. Then seeing a urine sample on the patient's bedside table, he dipped his finger in the sample and then touched his finger to his mouth, exclaiming that one can diagnose diabetes in this manner. All the students then dipped their finger into the urine and licked their finger. Osler scolded them: "If you would have observed carefully, I dipped my index finger into the urine and licked my little finger!" So much for careful observation— seemingly a lost art in medicine, preempted by ultrasound and imaging studies. Examining and interviewing patients in the traditional way has seemed to have disappeared, with physicians not engaging patients to assess them as unique and individual people and not laying on hands as physicians did in the past. I am referring specifically to inpatient rounds where the team enters the patient's room and no one touches and/or sits on the bed to interact with the patient.

Another story emphasizing history and physical examination occurred a few years ago when a resident presented a case to me of a child with exudative tonsillitis. Before entering the room, we discussed the differential diagnosis in order of what was most likely and what was treatable. When examining the patient, I noted edema of the upper eyelids and asked if the resident had noted this finding. She had not, and I suggested that the child had infectious mononucleosis based on this finding of Hoagland's sign. General Hoagland, a commandant at West Point in the 1950s, wrote a short booklet on infectious mononucleosis based on his experiences there and described upper eyelid edema in cadets with this disease. The fact is that nothing trumps a great history and physical exam, leading to 90% of diagnoses. Even if one didn't know that upper eyelid edema was associated with mononucleosis or classic trichinosis, such facts can be easily retrieved from iPhones and computers. There are so many other examples of these kinds of teaching tips that need to be passed on to trainees.

Lessons learned: The training one receives in history taking and physical diagnosis skills during medical school and residency is variable. In my generation, I became very well versed in many aspects of the history and physical, and recognized the importance of being expert in facilitating a reproducible and effective history and physical exam. At the Ohio State University in the 1960s, there was an emphasis on physical diagnosis skills, including mini-courses in ophthalmology and otolaryngology, with required reading of books authored by known department heads who oversaw these courses. It wasn't until I started seeing patients that I realized how important these courses would be in caring for my patients.

Using the framework of continuing professional development, we can all improve in how we provide patient care. One of the ways this can happen is through coaching (i.e., having a colleague sit in while you conduct part or all the exam). Atul Gawande's wonderful experience, as written in the *New Yorker* magazine (October 3, 2011), in which his former chair of surgery agreed to observe him (in essence, coach him) is an amazing example of a commitment to continued learning, even as a senior faculty member. We all can learn from examples like that and should push for adapting the same model in our own institutions. For example, most of us have been granted administrative time to complete medical records, write a grant, and collate information from colleagues for summative evaluations of trainees. Using this time to observe peers interacting with patients can be a valuable model for the division.

Coordinating this with leadership in medical education could lead to a study that would document the observations, using rigorous tools to do so.

I have observed how colleagues have developed expertise in caring for children with complex medical issues, psychosocial problems, and specific diagnoses (e.g., hyperactivity), as a few examples of ways to excel in patient care. For other specialties, there are parallel examples. Developing this expertise also mandates that you think about how you will measure the effectiveness of what you are doing. Documenting how you provide quality patient care can become a model for others to emulate and an objective activity that you can record in your educator portfolio.

TEACHING

The next area of focus for the junior CE is teaching, a role that seems to attract many physicians into academic medicine. Several important questions arise when thinking about teaching: How do I fit teaching in with a full patient care schedule? What knowledge and experience do I bring to the plate that will enable me to excel in teaching? Do I have sufficient content expertise with limited exposure to clinical patient care? What formal educational training have I had and how do I become an excellent teacher?

To answer the first question, we often think of teaching as a more formal session, such as a resident core lecture or a similar scenario for medical students. In actuality, CEs do most of their teaching on the fly, where there is no preparation and the content is specific and case-based. These are the situations where you need to understand adult learning principles and how to determine, based on the presentation and initial questioning, what knowledge and experience the learner has. I have always emphasized in my faculty development workshops that we should strive not to achieve a certain quantity of teaching but to teach consistently with each trainee interaction. There are times when we are inundated with patient care issues in the ambulatory, critical care, emergency, and inpatient units, thereby limiting the time we are able to teach. However, if you consider one or two teaching points when discussing each patient with trainees, you will be pleasantly surprised with feedback regarding your efforts. This can take less than a minute.

It is understandable that junior CEs have had limited experience in the clinical setting, which can create anxiety and reduced confidence in teaching. With each patient or trainee interaction, you will be reflecting on your own knowledge and experience, and assessing that of the trainee. Your overall goal, in my opinion, is to facilitate self-directed learning in residents and medical students, and that is accomplished by adhering to adult learning principles. As an example, assessing what their experience has been with each patient is a critical point in diagnosing the learner. Allowing them to provide you with their assessments of what they think is happening with the patient should become the focus of your teaching. So often I have not been certain of the patient's diagnosis and have, in concert with the trainee, delved into the literature to collect information that might lead to a diagnosis or at least a better understanding of the patient's problems.

Lastly, I have previously suggested that junior CEs negotiate for resources to attend faculty development sessions locally and/or nationally. Whereas virtual learning is also an alternative, for me, nothing takes the place of being physically present with peers and interacting with standardized learners as the ideal way to learn new skills and knowledge.

There are so many resources today as opposed to when I was a junior faculty member to help you teach more effectively. For example, I published a paper that involves the eight-step preceptor, a variation of the one-minute manager/preceptor (Ottolini et al. *Teach Learn Med.* 2010;22:97–101). Learning tips such as this allow teaching to happen on a regular basis, even if the teaching moments are brief. These stick with learners because they relate to the case they just saw (i.e., they are quite contextual). Some of us never receive formal teacher training in medical school or residency, even though today, there are numerous programs that teach medical students and residents how to teach, an area in which I have published extensively. In addition to case-based teaching in the ambulatory area, hospital, or emergency department, there are other teaching formats that junior faculty can explore to make teaching more effective.

Lecturing has been studied extensively and has not been effective in changing the behavior of participants, either regarding medical diagnoses and treatment or educational issues. That makes sense, as traditional lecturing is top-down (i.e., the teacher talking to passive learners). When you lecture in this format and view the audience (that is, when not focused on slides with your back to the audience), it is impossible to know where learners are in their knowledge and experience, and how they are connecting with the content of the lecture. As an alternative, interactive lecturing allows the teacher to assess learners, even in a large group. Yvonne Steinert from Montreal has published in this area and provides wonderful tips on how to engage large groups when you are expected to lecture. Another suggestion is to use the flipped classroom to activate learners outside the classroom so you can concentrate on higher cognitive thinking (Bloom's taxonomy) when interacting in person with the trainees. Addressing higher cognitive levels in the classroom allows participants to focus on the application of knowledge in the real world. Evaluating these classroom interactions is critical to assess their effectiveness and to document in your educator portfolio. It is commonplace in US medical schools and residency programs to use Likert scales to evaluate classroom educational activities. If you think about a recent lecture you have given, it was likely evaluated with a form using a Likert scale. We have all seen how trainees complete these forms (i.e., a straight line down the form for each question asked, incorporating all the 5s or 4s without any narrative). Sometimes limited discerning thought goes into the feedback forms that do not have narratives, leaving the CE with little information on what they did that was good and what needed correction. Over time, I have incorporated into my work Brookfield's Critical Incident Classroom Questionnaire, which comprises simple questions that enable learners to provide meaningful feedback. There are five questions: When were you most attracted in today's session? When were you most distanced? What surprised you most? What was most affirming? What did someone say that was most puzzling? I realize this takes more time for trainees to complete and not everyone is willing to complete the form. However, this data, analyzed qualitatively, provides great feedback that would not otherwise emerge with Likert scales. Brookfield presents a summary of the learners' comments the following class day, reaffirming that their feedback has been heard and processed. The teaching point here is that you don't have to depend on the institution's traditional Likert scale evaluation but can make Brookfield's evidence-based form or a modified version available for trainees to complete on their interactions with you. These narratives can be incorporated into educational scholarship projects, assessing trainee responses qualitatively. This is also how you can make an educator portfolio meaningful for individual growth and promotion purposes (i.e., documenting what you do as a CE). Even more importantly, if you can demonstrate that you have effected behavior change based on any of your activities, that is the bottom line. As I mentioned in the introduction and as part of the primer's title, bringing about change is the ultimate goal you should strive for in medical education.

Willie Sutton said he robbed banks because that's where the money is. It is easy to assume that improving one's teaching is where the money is. In fact, all teaching involves understanding the learner, the learning environment, the teacher, and the content to be taught. I suggest that before you focus on the characteristics of a great teacher, you need to study and apply adult learning theory, as emphasized by Malcolm Knowles, so as to understand how the learner approaches learning. This is a guide for searching for teaching excellence. Reading Knowles' work is ideal, but there are many review articles and commentaries that address adult learning that can provide the information you need to apply in a learning situation. I say this as I found it challenging not only to read about my pediatric patients but to also further my knowledge about education principles and applications. So, if you can find short-cuts in your reading, that may help you balance ongoing professional development in your specialty *and* in medical education. Some books in the annotated bibliography at the end of the primer can be helpful focused reading about specific educational issues, such as questioning skills.

There are a few summary comments about teaching that I think have been invaluable in my career. One is to make a conscious effort to teach tidbits of information on the fly that take seconds *but* give a message to trainees that you teach no matter what the circumstances. In the eight-step preceptorship that Ottolini and Greenberg have developed, an important step is to make a general teaching point. Announcing this with every patient (i.e., "I am going to make a teaching point") alerts the learners that a teaching point is coming. The same can be said for feedback, as it allows the trainee to first self-assess, and then you note what they have done well and what they can improve upon. In the end, you learn to adjust to every clinical situation but always commit to providing teaching and then feedback.

Several stories about teaching will illustrate my point. I vividly remember my last inpatient attending responsibility, which occurred before the advent of hospitalists. I had over 140 patients admitted to my service over the course of the month, and some of them were severely ill, like one newly diagnosed infant with Bruton's agammaglobulinemia and sepsis. Regularly scheduled one-hour teaching conferences were either totally eliminated or reduced to 30 minutes or less. Teaching during hospital rounds, or what we referred to as work rounds, was also limited because of the acuity of illness of our patients. I was feeling that trainees were being cheated because of the emphasis on patient care, understandably so. I would have liked to have taught more and had greater informal interactions with the students and residents. At the end of the difficult month on service, I received a beautiful note from the medical students thanking me profusely for my caring, modeling, and teaching. I had undervalued the teaching (brief but consistent), modeling, and humanistic characteristics I tried to convey, much of that occurring on work rounds, with and without discourse.

Here's a story involving the observation of trainees: As a junior CE, you might not have the same opportunities to observe trainees frequently, but when you do, there are things to think about. Over the last 18 years in my role as a part-time and voluntary attending physician, I have observed many students and even more residents as they interact with patients. I have often been asked by residents at the more senior level to observe and provide feedback on their counseling skills. On numerous occasions, I have done that and provided feedback that usually pertains to two areas. First is balancing the feedback talk by discussing the issues as interactively as possible (i.e., encouraging patient input and buy-in to the diagnosis and plan). Activating a patient or parent is no different than activating a learner. Second is making certain the patient or parent has not only heard what the resident has said but also committed to carrying it out. Following the feedback on this first resident-patient interaction, I seek to observe the same residents doing counseling again, obviously looking for behavior change based on my previous feedback. I have seen this change in behavior on the second and subsequent iterations, meaning that the residents not only have learned the information but have been able to apply it to the clinical setting. This closure of the learning loop is one of the most gratifying experiences a teacher can have. Knowing that you have effected change, perhaps forever in a positive way that will make patient care better, is as good as it gets. It addresses this statement: "I know when I am teaching. I need to know if you are learning." When you see it with your own eyes, it's magic.

Lessons learned: First, teaching and patient care go hand in hand and are basically inseparable. Trainees often do not demarcate when patient care is occurring versus when teaching occurs. The only way this division can be clearer in the learner's mind is for teachers to announce when they make a teaching point. This will help to separate these two areas and alert learners that teaching or learning is happening. This teaching around patients illustrates the adult learning principle of the importance of context, which allows learners to retain the information more effectively. Second, we can't always teach in formal settings the way we planned because of patient care demands. Teaching in snippets every day and consistently resonates with trainees, and they appreciate that effort.

In addition, I found that attending national and regional Association of American Medical Colleges meetings and networking with educators from many schools enhanced my career educationally, more so than if I had only networked with peers in my own specialty. I owe a debt of gratitude to those earning advanced degrees in education, as they have taught me so much and have enhanced my teaching and educational scholarship. I have anecdotally observed that most of my peers have not taken this same route and, nonetheless, have become leaders in education. Importantly, specialties have been the focus of CEs developing their educational expertise, unlike when I started my career. This growth of CEs assuming the major responsibility for teaching and educational scholarship has enabled them to share ideas and research with one another in their specialties. I am not suggesting that national educational groups, like the Association of American Medical Colleges, are passé, just that there may be less of a need for them as education has flourished in specialties. Whichever path one takes, make education a focus of your continuing professional development since these are the activities in which CEs are involved every day.

EDUCATIONAL SCHOLARSHIP

I would now like to segue to another important part of the mission statement of academic health centers; i.e., educational scholarship. Educational scholarship is distinguished from traditional research in that CEs are challenged to study new innovations they implement in order to make certain that they are effective and evidence-based. Very early into a career as a CE, finding time to do educational scholarship is a significant task to confront. Getting your feet on the ground in terms of meeting colleagues and trainees, developing a cohort of patients, understanding the computer system in place for the institution in general and for the electronic medical record, creating a schedule for conferences, and learning where the bathrooms are represent formidable tasks you need to accomplish before thinking about educational scholarship. With time, these issues will be old hand, and at some point, you need to consider what kind of educational scholarship you want to do. Some faculty will have had research experience in a previous job or as a medical student, resident, or fellow. If the content area of a previous study was one that you felt inspired by and want to pursue, that would be a natural option. If there are no specific areas of education that you are interested in pursuing, let me suggest that many topics that we take for granted have not been studied, or if they have, there are additional aspects of that topic needing further study. These areas for study are literally things we encounter every day; questioning whether they are evidence-based can lead to educational scholarship.

You can choose to start a project or study de novo, or can explore what fellow faculty are doing in educational scholarship and whether there is the possibility of collaborating. This might be an opportunity to discuss your interests with your division chief and determine if the chief knows of faculty studying a specific content area. Even if unaware of ongoing studies, he or she may be able to guide you to faculty with this information, such as the head of the appointment, promotion, and tenure committee; the chair of your specialty; the head of faculty affairs; or the chair of the institutional review board. Hooking onto other faculty's research as you start your new job is a great path to take, assuming there is something of interest to you and the time involvement is reasonable.

At this point in your career, I suggest you consider collaborating with others for many reasons. First and most important, collaborating will link you with fellow faculty, hopefully those at the mid or senior level, who have had publication experience and bring different strengths to the plate. Second, seeking collaborators with similar interests will enable you to establish ongoing scholarship over time, building on what you and others have previously done. Third, getting started in educational scholarship where responsibilities are shared with others makes the possibility of bringing a project to closure more likely as opposed to working by yourself. Sharing the responsibilities for developing a study, gathering data, analyzing that data, and writing conclusions makes your job easier than doing it alone.

I've seen how caring mid-level and senior-level CEs can reach out and engage junior CEs in scholarship. A few years ago, our general pediatric department hired a new faculty member whose main job was patient care in the ambulatory area, although she did have expertise in adolescent birth control and would develop that interest in her short stay at Children's. I was volunteering and observing residents there and frequently made small talk with her about life, family, professional goals, and so forth. A few months into her employment, I asked if she might be interested in doing educational scholarship together on observing residents' communication skills. She was interested, and I suggested we enlist three medical students to be part of our team to perform the observation part of the study. The benefits for the students would be for them to see how residents work with patients, be coauthors on the study, and learn about methodology, research design, and evaluation. That study indeed happened, not without some glitches, but we completed it and finally had it accepted by a reputable journal. In addition, since we needed statistical help, we also invited a statistician from George Washington University to be a coauthor. I was able to observe this junior CE organize and take control of the study, delegating responsibilities appropriately to the medical students working with us. I initially provided her with some key articles on the topic, which became the basis for the study question: Do residents ask about parents' main concern in an acute care visit and determine why that concerns them? I was very impressed with her work ethic and ability to complete the project in a timely fashion despite the usual barriers in educational scholarship one encounters along the way.

Lessons learned: This story illustrates a number of important teaching points when doing educational scholarship. If you are lucky, a more senior-level CE might reach out to you to do collaborative research. If the content area to be studied is interesting to you, grab the opportunity. Make certain you ask questions along the way to clarify and define any questions you have about the study and what your perceived role will be. The next lesson is that engaging medical students or college students (if they are available) to carry out responsibilities in a study—like in this case, observing residents interviewing parents—is critical in nonfunded studies. Basically, while you are seeing patients, the medical students are concomitantly collecting data for the study. They also can be helpful in entering data, and one student with whom I worked actually performed the statistical analysis on a paper recently accepted for publication. Many students have served as coauthors on my studies, and in most cases, they are first authors. When engaging medical students *and* junior CEs, I prefer that the latter be first author, as junior CEs need first authorship for eventual promotion. Different members of the team can be first authors for different aspects of the study (e.g., a student can be first author on an abstract submitted to a meeting and the junior CE on the paper).

I also have included many residents on my papers. This happens in a number of ways. First, residents seek me out because they know of my educational interests. Second, when the content of the study involves residents—like residents as teachers using the flipped classroom technique—it is strategically wise to involve individuals who might be influential in convincing colleagues of the study's importance. Third, residents seek mentoring for projects they are doing as part of the requirements for their training.

Another lesson I learned early in my career is that my area of expertise is not statistics. On the paper I mentioned earlier involving resident communication skills, we invited a statistician from George Washington University to help with this work and invited her to be a coauthor. Over the years, there have been many statisticians at Children's and George

Washington University that have contributed to my studies and have been coauthors on my publications.

I present an interesting story about how educational scholarship can evolve de novo through conversations with colleagues. Almost 40 years ago, a colleague in hematology-oncology said she was working on a national curriculum for residents in pediatric oncology and asked if I was aware of any literature on residents giving patients bad news around the diagnosis of acute lymphocytic leukemia. My initial reaction was that it was unethical for residents to be informing parents that their child has cancer without training in this area and supervision. My second response was that I was not aware of any curriculum that addressed that issue, and I asked if she was interested in collaborating on a study to assess how residents give bad news. In short, we developed an innovative curriculum using standardized parents in which second-year pediatric residents had to inform these parents that their child had acute lymphocytic leukemia. We actually recruited parents who had a child diagnosed with leukemia, knowing they had worked through the difficult psychosocial issues associated with this life-threatening diagnosis. We trained them on two case scenarios, teaching them their role in each case and the importance of their staying in role while receiving the diagnosis. Interestingly, a number of parents reflected on when they received this life-altering diagnosis and recalled that the experience with the informing physician was not always positive. On the residents' first interaction with the parents, we taught the parents to give the residents feedback using standardized forms we developed to document essential content issues and communication skills. Two weeks later, the residents had to do a similar exercise with a second set of parents, having received feedback after their first iteration. We postulated that there would be short-term improvement in both content and communication skills. As predicted, their short-term skills and content improved, and the study was published in 1982 (Jewett, Greenberg et al. *Ped* 1982;70:907–911), 40 years ago. It is clear that educational scholarship ideas are present every day in one's workplace. The questioning of things we have accepted for generations and not studied can lead to educational scholarship and make significant contributions to the literature. Even established studies can have gaps not addressed that make for important scholarship.

Again, at this level of a CE, you are not as likely to be the originator of educational scholarship as when you reach mid-level status. You have many competing responsibilities that will consume your time, especially patient care. Joining others in their scholarship is ideal, only if you are interested in the content area involved. Also, being a team player in these efforts is important, but it is also important to avoid overextending yourself. When projects are envisioned to create numerous publication possibilities (abstracts, more than one article), negotiating first authorship on one of those possibilities is important before you start the data collection or the literature review.

Another issue is whether to approach educational scholarship broadly, as I did, or focus on a particular aspect as your career evolves. There is no right or wrong answer, and perhaps the most helpful comment I can make is to follow your passion. I loved doing all the educational scholarship I was involved in, and this opened new horizons for me. Nearly all, if not all, of what I published became a part of my educational persona. Most of what I studied was translatable into clinical practice and immediately applicable to improve clinicians' patient care and educational responsibilities. What comes to mind are empathy, communication skills, teaching how to teach, learner issues, and change in the way we have traditionally done things, like lecturing. Although I didn't see myself focusing on a particular area of education, themes emerged that received most of my attention: communication and teaching skills.

What is critical for CEs is to document what they do in any of their activities, and this is usually done in an educator portfolio, recognized by many medical schools as an important tool to record CE activities for promotion purposes. The portfolio format can follow what might be used locally in the department or medical school, or can follow published examples, such as those available online from the Medical College of Wisconsin. A warning is that it is not enough to just list activities one participates in, as this does not provide any insight on the quality of those endeavors. An example I frequently encounter in reviewing curricula vitae is a listing of teaching experiences. When I see this, my question is always "So what difference did your teaching make in each of these cases, and how did you document that?" The important learning point is that the onus is on you to provide evidence that what you do has made a difference in patient care, educational scholarship, teaching, and advocacy.

ADVOCACY

Advocacy is a major part of the academic health center mission statement for pediatrics but not necessarily for other specialties. That is not to say that advocacy is not needed across specialties. In pediatrics, faculty speak on behalf of children whose voices may not be heard since they are too young to vote and have no voice for themselves. Getting families good housing free of lead and vermin, clean water, bicycle helmets, infant car seats, and other preventive health measures are examples of advocacy in which CEs can be involved. There are many other examples, such as securing home health care for families with a child with disabilities, guaranteeing access to healthy food in areas where there are food deserts, and seeking financial help when a child's health is at stake. In other specialties, CEs can also advocate for patients through housing for the homeless or new immigrants, coordinating multidisciplinary care, ensuring and being cognizant that lower socioeconomic patients get care similar to that of those more entitled, and making certain there are resources for elderly people living alone. Other areas of advocacy are through patient education, involvement in the political arena by educating politicians about the dangers to health and the importance of health maintenance, and involvement in national organizations that influence decision-making about health. Advocating for those who are less fortunate or without a voice can be a very important part of patient care. Again, documenting one's efforts and how these impacted patients is important when it comes to promotion on the academic ladder.

MENTORING

A topic that stands alone from educational scholarship, teaching, and patient care is mentoring. It is critical to align yourself with mentors when starting your career so that others can understand your career goals and support you. Mentors can play different roles in your career so that one mentor for some faculty will not fill all needs. I see mentors as faculty available within and outside your institution. Your first mentor as a junior faculty member will most likely come from within the institution. As you become more active nationally, seeking mentors from those sources is more logical.

So, what kind of mentor is beneficial? I always consider gender issues when thinking about mentoring. With so many younger women represented in medicine, it can be useful for a woman who is a junior CE to seek out a mid-level or senior-level female CE. Issues that might arise are balancing professional and work life, timing of pregnancy, seeking the same remuneration that men in the same position receive, working your way up the promotion ladder, dealing with gender issues that unfortunately are ingrained in academic medicine (e.g., sexual and verbal harassment), getting involved in educational scholarship, attaining leadership positions, and other similar life and professional topics. In some instances, that same mentor might also have expertise in many areas and could be the only mentor you need.

Other mentors may be chosen specifically because they are role models who have established themselves in specific parts of the academic health center's mission, like educational scholarship. Again, such a person could be from one's own institution or university setting. In my career, I have collaborated with faculty from the Kellogg Business School at Northwestern; faculty from the GWU Graduate School of Education and Human Development; a linguist at the National Institutes of Health; faculty at numerous medical schools; pediatric clerkship directors from around the country; the creators of *Lion in the House* (2007 Emmy winner for Best Nonfiction Documentary); faculty in physical therapy; and physician assistants, obstetricians, neurosurgeons, psychiatrists, hospital medicine, neurologists, anesthesiologists, internists, and statisticians, most at George Washington University. The point is that over time, I have engaged faculty from other disciplines, and occasionally from outside of medicine, providing me a large pool from which to choose a mentor. In essence, my own mentors have represented pediatrics and the field of medical education.

As junior CEs, it is likely you would choose a mentor based on your early work experiences and faculty with whom you are in contact. It can take time for junior CEs to get to know mid- and senior-level CEs. In that period, you can speak with a division chair or colleague about issues and questions. You can be proactive by thinking about areas that need to be addressed, some that may be gaps, and others where you need confirmation that you are on track to success. Specifying what you want from a mentor is also important as you try to align your interests with those who would mentor you. Your mission statement will be important here as you describe to a would-be mentor what you stand for as a CE. Finally, mentor relationships can change over time as you ascend the promotion ladder and acquire more experience.

Lessons learned: Develop a relationship with a more experienced faculty member to have frank discussions on topics of personal and professional importance. Whereas others' experiences may not be applicable to your specific situation, having an experienced CE listen to your thought processes and raise questions for clarification, along with probing questions that further elucidate how you are thinking, can be comforting and confirming. Mentors who understand us as professionals and human beings can push us further than we ever thought we could be pushed. These become people who believe in us and who feel a vested interest in our success and well-being. Many become lifelong friends, extending well beyond their roles as mentors in our personal and professional lives. They are there for us when we have family life cycle celebrations in addition to when we suffer loss. Many become an integral part of our being.

ADMINISTRATIVE RESPONSIBILITIES AND LEADERSHIP

I now want to segue to an area for which few of us have trained and which many of us see as a necessary evil in carrying out the mission of the academic health center: the administrative responsibilities that come with the job. It is a poor commentary that few of us in academic medicine have been taught how to run a meeting, develop a strategic plan, or lead a brainstorming session to make decisions on important areas. Again, it is not uncommon for you as junior CEs to be selected for an important position within the department, such as clerkship director or resident training program director. While that is certainly flattering and implies a sense of trust and confidence in your abilities, it also comes with significant responsibilities that may be foreign in your career due to lack of experience. So again, there are some important things to think about when considering this career option: How does it fit with your mission statement? What skills and knowledge do you have that will enable you to be successful in this job? What skills and knowledge are lacking that are essential to do this job correctly? What is the commitment of the department to support you in this endeavor (e.g., providing an appropriate budget and administrative support; funding you to advance your educational and leadership needs; and making the roles, responsibilities, and expectations of the job transparent)? What is the appropriate percentage of time commitment to the job to allow you to function effectively without negatively affecting your other roles and responsibilities? How will this position enable you to climb the promotional ladder, understanding that your patient care and/or educational scholarship time might be minimized? Ideally, you would be groomed for a significant position, like clerkship or residency director, through an assistant position, and then you would work your way up. The downside of taking an assistant's position is that the current clerkship and residency directors may elect to stay in place a long time, limiting your upward mobility at your institution.

Of course, there are many other administrative positions that are readily available in the division, the department, and the medical school. Chairing committees and completing mandated activities, like quality assurance, represent areas in which you can assume leadership, depending on your interests and mission statement. If quality assurance is an area you want to focus on, showing interest in it can lead to leadership positions—perhaps not immediately but a few years into your tenure with the division. If you become an assistant clerkship or residency director, again more likely after a few years at the center, you will automatically become a member of these committees that meet at least monthly regarding residents and medical students. Serving on committees provides some insight into the workings of different areas and also highlights the political climate at any center (i.e., the power structure within the institution, the preparedness of committee chairs and members to conduct important business, the efficiency of meetings, and how necessary change is effected in medicine).

In your own educator portfolio, it is not enough to list what committees you served on and chaired. This list can be boring to read when promotion decisions are made versus providing a narrative on how you contributed to the committees on which you served. As an example, suggesting an innovation that was adopted by a committee would be an important area to list in your portfolio. Another suggestion is making a seamless pathway evident to all regarding how decisions made in a committee progress to the department's executive committee and then on to the board of trustees of the institution.

Lessons learned: Once you start to acclimate to your new job over time (and that period can differ from faculty member to faculty member), it is reasonable to think about how you want to expand your horizons within the division, the department, or the medical school through committee work and/or mandated areas, such as overseeing quality assurance. This will help to build your educator portfolio early on and establish a path to promotion, which in essence is recognition by peers that you have been successful. A logical progression is to accept a committee assignment that best fits with your mission statement and career plan. This would be ideal but is not always realistic. So, selecting a committee that sounds interesting and that might increase the depth and breadth of your early professional life is a reasonable option. Perhaps it is a committee that deals with patient care or education, either of which might be in sync with your mission statement. As a new member of a committee, you will be learning how the committee functions, who makes up the membership, and what political nuances occur during and outside of meetings. Once you learn the lay of the land, you can decide how you want to contribute to the group and think about how you will document your contributions through your educator portfolio. An important role of an effective committee member is to ask provocative questions that may challenge the norms and what has been accepted without evidence.

CONCLUSION

The many lessons learned as a junior CE have been enumerated to provide some suggestions and lessons learned based on my experiences. Since my professional career evolved in another era, not all my comments will be pertinent to junior faculty starting their careers as CEs. However, until recently, I have occasionally written letters of recommendation for faculty I have known over the years. Reading their CVs informs me of their accomplishments and what I see as gaps that they have omitted. Converting long laundry lists of activities, such as lectures, committee participation, and collaborative ventures, into details about the impact you have made with patients, trainees, and colleagues will be the ticket to recognition by peers.

So, after thinking about your personal mission statement upon entering the academic world, what will be your major focus for the first five years? Whichever area you choose, developing a game plan (strategic plan, if you will) with timelines is a great idea. Most important is visualizing how your educator portfolio is going to look based on the area(s) you choose as your focus. No decision you make regarding your career is irrevocable and always subject to change. Experiencing different areas and keeping an open mind about new ventures can actually lead to a eureka moment when you find something that resonates and seems natural for you to do, at least in the short term. Although I had no formal research background or understanding of the nuances that comprise educational scholarship, I learned from others and involved faculty in my studies who not only enhanced the specific study but also allowed me to grow professionally through their role-modeling, mentoring, and sharing of their knowledge.

3

The Mid-Level Clinician Educator

When does one graduate from a junior to a mid-level clinician educator (CE)? I assume the answer is in the eyes of the beholder, but I would suggest that once one becomes eligible for promotion to associate professor, one graduates to the next CE level. In my view, this occurs at a range of 6 to 20 years after starting one's career, depending on academic achievements, with many faculty having built an educator portfolio worthy of promotion much closer to six to eight years after the start of an academic career. A major factor that pushes the timeline further out for promotion is the biologic clock for women in medicine who seek to have children. Studies have demonstrated that women are promoted to this level and the next significantly later than men because women choose to have children during a time when they would be productive in educational scholarship and other parts of the mission. It is hoped that chairs of divisions and departments understand this factor as a major reason for decreased educational scholarship compared to men at the same age. That is not to say that women shouldn't strive to maximally build their portfolio before bearing children and then resume their efforts after rejoining the workforce, in whatever capacity.

That said, this might be a good time for mid-level CEs to relook at their mission statement to determine if it needs revising based on new opportunities and responsibilities, both within and outside the medical center. As your career advances and opportunities present themselves at a leadership level or with collaboration around scholarship, these factors can change what a mission statement looks like. Again, using that mission statement as a way to define yourself professionally is a helpful guide to what you want to do versus what others see you doing.

DOI: 10.1201/9781003296270-3

This brief story illustrates how a mission statement can help in difficult decision-making. At some point later in my career as a mid-level CE, I was offered a position on the board of a national pharmacist association. The responsibilities as board member were presented to me, and the time involvement was not major, but it was significant. Although I was flattered by the offer, looking at my mission statement and the responsibilities I had, I informed my contact person that this would not work out for me. In retrospect, it was the correct decision based on where I saw my career path progressing at the time. The ability to say no is an important part of being satisfied with one's work, having life-work balance, and staying true to one's mission statement. Of course, you might feel emotionally that you let someone down by saying no, but there are other ways you can demonstrate that you are a team player.

PATIENT CARE

Patient care is likely to remain the number one priority at this stage, and further developing your expertise in this area is important. Some faculty develop a focus on patients presenting with complex problems, while others might find poorly diagnosed or documented problems as an area in which to develop expertise. Those with specialty training beyond that of a generalist have many options within their field and can concentrate efforts around a particular aspect of that field. I have a cardiology colleague at Children's who has done some exciting and groundbreaking work on teaching residents about referrals to cardiology when dealing with frequent diagnoses, such as syncope and chest pain. The work he has done focuses on the importance of making the decision to refer or not, based on details of the patient's presenting problem. In one scenario regarding syncope, there is a need for immediate referral because of a potentially life-threatening arrhythmia being the most likely diagnosis. The other scenario does not warrant referral but focuses more on hydration with exercise. In both cases, there is a need for effective communication with the patient or parents, which he included in his study. He has published a series of articles on teaching the referral process to trainees as his area of interest.

Generalists may have a specific interest in their field (e.g., lipid metabolism) and become the go-to person in the division when questions arise about that topic. Other generalists may enjoy all aspects of patient care and do not choose to emphasize a specific area of their practice.

A story can illustrate how focusing on a particular diagnosis or problem can enhance one's patient care and teaching activities at the same time. For years, I was fascinated with how poorly pediatricians diagnose middle ear diseases in children. In my medical school training, otolaryngology was emphasized, and I learned about middle ear disease, knowing I was likely choosing pediatrics as a career. As a junior CE, I read extensively about the different manifestations of middle ear disease and learned with on-the-job training how to diagnose different disorders, some requiring antibiotic therapy and others requiring watchful waiting and occasional referral to otolaryngology for surgical intervention. The real problem I noted was that faculty were not teaching the physical diagnosis skills of the middle ear adequately, meaning that many patients were being treated unnecessarily with antibiotics for effusions in the middle ear instead of required watchful waiting. Teaching residents as part of the physical exam how to adequately restrain a patient who was not willing or able to cooperate with the nonpainful exam was one of the first teaching points. Placing toddlers and preschool children in a prone position on their abdomen allows for easy restraining by the accompanying parent, who firmly holds the child's hands at the small of the back. The physician is then able to gently hold down the patient's head with one hand and examine the ear with the other, allowing for adequate visualization of the tympanic membrane. Then the exam itself requires knowledge of the tympanic membrane structures and how to use a pneumatic otoscope. If trainees have some understanding of the dynamics of middle ear physiology, then teaching them to recognize the position of the tympanic membrane can be key to making correct diagnoses about middle ear disease. The use of the pneumatic otoscope basically substantiates what one sees when examining the tympanic membrane (i.e., if the drum is retracted); then blowing air into it (positive pressure) will not move it, but withdrawing air will cause it to move to its neutral position. Thus, teaching a physical diagnosis skill like this can help ensure more accurate diagnoses in the future and reduce the overuse of antibiotics. Having residents call for your input on patients with middle ear disease helps to substantiate how well they have learned the physical exam nuances of the spectrum of those problems, from a normal tympanic membrane to one that is infected. Your confirming or denying their assessment can be an impactful teaching point that carries over into practice for them. Their feedback on how you assisted them to make accurate diagnoses of the middle ear can be incorporated into the educator portfolio.

Other physical exam maneuvers learned with time include reducing a nursemaid's elbow, recognizing the association between a bifid uvula and a submucous cleft palate, doing a cover/uncover eye test to detect a phoria or tropia, and recognizing an undescended testicle by observation and not palpation. Of course, these are all examples from my pediatrics experience, and those in other specialties can identify similar maneuvers or observations in their area of expertise. Teaching these skills to trainees perpetuates the art of medicine associated with patient care, and hopefully, those trainees will pass these skills down to the next generation.

Another story about patient care at mid-career involves directly observing trainees and providing feedback to them based on what you see. An example is a story about a neonatology fellow at our institution who was a wonderful resident and continued to see her continuity patients even into her fellowship. I asked if I could observe her one afternoon as she was going to see a patient and family that she had known for over three years. In that encounter, I noted that, in the room, there were the mother and three children, one of whom was the patient. All the seats were occupied, so the fellow chose to stand during the interview. When we exited the room and found time to debrief, I asked her what she thought of the encounter in general. I followed that question by asking her why she decided to stand. She immediately saw where I was going with this questioning and recognized she was not sitting during the encounter. I asked why, and she responded that all the seats in the room were occupied. I asked her, in retrospect, to problem-solve that fact, and she came up with an alternative so that she could be sitting. We further discussed how standing instead of sitting could imply a power differential and diminish the voice of the patient. It can also contribute to trust issues and lead to the patient's nonadherence to medical advice because of problems with developing a mutual relationship. I don't think this former trainee will ever forget that scenario. These critical incidents that occur often impact trainees, and they can remember information like that their entire careers.

Lessons learned: As one becomes a mid-level CE, fine-tuning physical diagnosis and observation skills is a great way to enhance patient care, as are handoff skills and impartment of knowledge to trainees in the context of the art of medicine. As mentioned previously, combining patient care with teaching is like BOGO: buy one, get one free. It is so important that mid-level and senior CEs focus on aspects of patient care as we train our future physicians. I prided myself on my knowledge and skills of middle ear disease, where I was the go-to faculty person when there were questions. I not only understood the anatomy and pathophysiology of the middle ear, I knew how to apply that knowledge and skill for the patient. I found that none of my colleagues used the pneumatic otoscope and that, invariably, when a trainee called me to assess a child with middle ear disease, their assessment was incorrect more than 80% to 90% of the time. That informed me we were not teaching this properly. Therefore, I encouraged trainees to let me verify their diagnoses around middle ear issues so that I could instruct them about the pathophysiology of the tympanic membrane and middle ear pressures, and how that affected what the tympanic membrane looked like.

It goes without saying that teaching the long-held, traditional bedside or chairside aspects of the physical exam is important. Percussing a chest or abdomen, properly palpating an abdomen when you suspect organomegaly, assessing bowel sounds, and observing nailbeds and mucous membranes for color are all physical diagnosis procedures that have become a lost art in medicine. The art of interviewing is also important to teach, such as giving positive affirmation, determining the main concern of the patient, stating in specific terms that the patient is not alone in dealing with a problem, and establishing trust and rapport are all critical incidents to teach future caregivers.

TEACHING

Enhancing teaching skills should be a priority at this stage, being creative and looking for new ways to teach principles of a particular topic and, at the same time, studying any new technique to assess its efficacy. These techniques may emanate from participating in workshops nationally and at the medical center, reading articles and books on education and leadership, speaking with colleagues about their experiences, and questioning shibboleths handed down from generation to generation that have not been studied. As I have stated elsewhere, it is important for the promotion process to document the impact of your teaching. Without repeating what I have suggested for entry-level CEs, I am going to illustrate my point with a couple of poignant stories.

The first story focuses on what other disciplines can teach us about certain issues. I was at an international medical education meeting and heard a seasoned and well-respected surgeon from Great Britain discuss how he sought out an expert seamstress to watch her work and determine if there were tips he could adapt to suturing in his surgical practice. He went on to explain how this experience impacted his practice. I wondered at the time if there were other examples that could be adapted to benefit medicine. This thinking evolved into writing a commentary in collaboration with a colleague about how jazz groups can inform better communication for those delivering interdisciplinary care to complex patients. We described how accomplished jazz ensembles (e.g., trios, quartets, quintets, and sextets) work together harmoniously, despite many instances of improvisation, changes in the leadership of a group, and songs that are arranged for a specific instrument as examples (Pearl and Greenberg, *Med Teach.* 2020;42:1337–1342). Jazz musicians talk to each other on every song, picking up cues from body language and where the melody is heading. They have no problem with who leads on each musical piece they play, and each musician strives not only to excel individually but to play with others in the group as if they were one. Another example of how team members function effectively outside of medicine is the Blue Angels. They were featured in a History Channel documentary, and what was significant about their approach to flying 18 inches apart wing tip to wing tip was their intensive preparation for each flyover. They spoke in detail about how to respond to commands and how their roles evolved in this amazing and coordinated endeavor. No room for error here.

We postulated that interprofessional groups could learn important principles from how other disciplines work in harmony. There is so much to learn from other disciplines if we take our blinders off and think more creatively. Another collaboration with a faculty member of the Kellogg School of Business at Northwestern University resulted in a paper we published on perspective taking, a technique that promotes putting yourself in the shoes of the client or patient when making business or medical decisions.

The second story starts with an abstract in 1999 and how this resulted in a model on how to observe trainees in the clinical setting. The model proposed by this abstract, called brief structured observation, focused on observing a trainee for three to five minutes, writing down everything the trainee said, and then providing the trainee with timely and objective feedback after the observation. Unfortunately, the authors, Pituch et al. (1999), never either studied or published their work beyond the abstract. That is where the scholarship of application, as noted by Glassick and Boyer in their seminal books, makes an appearance. I realized the potential power of this observation model and, over time, in the early 2000s, built upon and edited the model for the ambulatory setting by incorporating ground rules for the setting up of the observation, the time spent observing and what the faculty member was to do in the room, and the feedback process following the observation, both oral and written. This important model conveys to faculty that they can observe a trainee and provide feedback connected to the Accreditation Council for Graduate Medical Education milestones in less than ten minutes. I have presented the model at academic centers as part of a visiting professorship, and the feedback from participants (clinical faculty) has been very positive, with an undetermined number using the model in their own settings. In combining teaching with scholarship, I published this paper in 2021 with a George Washington University medical student and valued colleague from Children's Hospital. Of course, it is sometimes difficult to have a nice delineated border between teaching, patient care, and educational scholarship, but they do and should, indeed, blend on many occasions.

It was at this mid-level stage and beyond that I was most involved with visiting professorships in medical education and was also honored to speak at three universities, addressing faculty in different fields, such as law, humanities, and business. As you network nationally and develop a community of learners, you are likely to be invited to speak, and it is a wonderful opportunity to advocate for your areas of interest. Three areas I often discussed during visiting professorships were case-based teaching, diagnosing and dealing with the problem learner, and observing trainees in their interactions with patients. I have published in two of those areas, and the problem learner workshop entailed having a medical student portray a problem learner based on a real-life situation that evolved into an interesting outcome.

Another area that became an important part of my professional career was developing workshops that combined evidence-based information and practice. These fall under the heading of faculty development. Almost all the workshops I facilitated were created de novo, with some knowledge and skills incorporated from other educational sessions I attended. The important aspect of these workshops, in my opinion, was to make certain there were practice opportunities for participants to translate knowledge into practice. That principle stimulated and challenged me to think about the flipped classroom as a technique in workshops, allowing for more time for hands-on practice. Segueing into faculty development sessions felt most natural when I was confident about content and application around a specific topic. I conducted workshops locally and nationally, collaborating with colleagues who added another perspective to the workshops. Interacting with seasoned participants also afforded me new knowledge and experiences. In more than one occasion when I attended a workshop at national meetings, facilitators asked, "Why are you here? You are the expert?" My response, humbly, was always that there was much for me to learn from other perspectives, information that enriched my knowledge and inspired me to go down paths I had not considered.

As an example of the workshops and innovative curricula that evolved, a students-as-teachers course as a fourth-year elective at George Washington University was created by my colleague and myself in 1995 and is still going strong. It might be the longest and most studied program like this in the country. As many as half of the senior class elect to take this course, which traverses their senior year. We developed workshops around adult learning principles and their applications, teaching a skill, feedback, and case-based teaching. Each workshop presented underlying content or principles as pre-class preparation reading, and in class, we spent time focusing on performance or behavior. At the outset of this course, we realized there was too much teacher and not enough learner talk, so we revised the workshops and made them more learner-centered in concert with adult learning theory.

Lessons learned: Facilitating workshops allows one to reinforce educational principles, impart new knowledge and skills to fellow faculty and trainees, collaborate with faculty nationally who have similar interests, and inform colleagues about your interests. The content of many of these workshops resulted in educational scholarship over time. In addition, as one builds an educator portfolio, having workshops accepted in a peer review process for national meetings allows one to include these activities in the portfolio.

Creative CEs often think out of the box and develop new teaching techniques that can potentially make an impact on trainee learning. I don't want to be redundant, but any innovation that one creates can be transformed into educational scholarship by thinking about how to measure the effectiveness of the program. I have always suggested that once you develop goals and objectives, think about the evaluation, which often determines the methods you use to assess the program's effectiveness. Since some educational scholarships I created are not tried-and-true randomized controlled studies, there are other ways to measure the effectiveness of an intervention. Using the brief structured observation model described earlier, I knew that the feedback in workshops I facilitated and from residents with whom I interacted on the model would contribute to my outcome measures. This concept is so important, as I have heard from my many interactions nationally with CE colleagues of wonderful teaching techniques without rigorous measurements of outcomes. It is a simple mantra for me: Most of the time that I developed an educational innovation, I thought about outcomes first and how I would measure them. The exceptions occurred when I was a junior CE and hadn't thought about that concept and the importance of translating teaching into educational scholarship.

EDUCATIONAL SCHOLARSHIP

Educational scholarship, if this is the focus for a CE, should peak mid-career as one approaches the professor level on the academic ladder. I found that doing educational scholarship at this stage was mostly collaborative, reaching out to residents, medical students, allied health faculty, and fellow faculty. There were also many examples of collaboration at the national level, performing multi-institutional research. As noted earlier about collaborations in educational scholarship over time, I looked for partnerships with faculty from other disciplines, both within and outside of medicine. There are faculty in your specialty, other specialties, and across disciplines who have a passion for education and might be waiting for you to approach them about a curricular innovation or educational scholarship study. These partnerships don't happen unless you go out of your comfort zone and contact others about your interests. Sometimes you find like-minded people when you see references you cite in a study you have done; sometimes it's through small talk at a national meeting or someone coming to a workshop you have facilitated (or vice versa) where you quickly see what you have in common. This was how I met Margaret Plack, PhD, EdD, a superb physical therapist, educator, and researcher, who coauthored an article with me on reflection, which was published in *Pediatrics* in 2005. It is the most cited article I have written, with more than 215 citations. She and I have conducted numerous national workshops together on reflection and have published a number of articles on assessing reflective practice.

Having others take the lead in educational scholarship with you overseeing their efforts requires another skill set. Instead of you taking charge and running full steam ahead, you are more in a consultative role, watching how plans unfold. What is critical is that those assuming major responsibility for a project have a game plan and timeline from the start to the end, with you making certain that they adhere to these timelines. In essence, you become somewhat of a benevolent task master and available for any issues or questions that arise. In addition, in terms of authorship, if you are the lead in the educational scholarship and have not achieved the professorial rank, you need to be first author. On the other hand, if you have attained full professorship, you may consider being the last author, the most senior. That happened quite frequently in the more senior part of my career, with medical students and residents being first authors, despite the fact that all the educational scholarship with trainees have been the result of my creation.

Here's a poignant story to illustrate the point about how educational scholarship can evolve from discussions with colleagues. A mid-level CE in a subspecialty division of pediatrics came to me and voiced concern that she was unable to change resident behavior with patients around a very important area. She further related that she was assigned five sessions with the residents during their core lecture series to present the essential information around this common problem in pediatrics. In our conversation, I inquired what content she was delivering and how she imparted that content during those sessions. She replied that the five sessions were all traditional lectures followed by a Q and A period. She assumed that the content she was providing could have resulted in resident behavior change based on the importance of the information and the fact that residents commonly cared for patients with this diagnosis. However, there was one problem: there are many evidence-based articles in the literature confirming that top-down lectures do not result in behavior change, whether regarding medical care or educational issues. I introduced her to the concept of the interactive lecture and adult learning principles through some relatively short and basic readings on the topics. She totally changed how she delivered this information to the residents, using interactive and learner-centered responses as opposed to her lecture format. As a way to assess resident understanding and performance following these five sessions, residents experienced an inpatient rotation where they encountered patients as described in her sessions. Based on the intervention she developed in one of the sessions, she measured resident behavior around caring for inpatients on this rotation, noting marked increases in improvement in patient care after the intervention. This evolved into a quality assurance project and resulted in two papers citing this patient care improvement following the learner-centered sessions. So, this was a major success story on four accounts: (1) it contributed to the faculty member's understanding of adult learning theory and interactive lecturing, (2) it addressed patient care through quality assurance, (3) it resulted in educational scholarship, and (4) it improved teaching with the residents. Now, the result of that kind of curricular innovation is the penultimate in outcomes (i.e., impacting patient care) and doesn't happen very often as documented in the literature.

Lessons learned: In terms of educational scholarship, my advice to mid-level CEs depends on their academic level. If you have achieved the professor level, it is time to be the idea person and hand off studies to more junior people and trainees, while remaining available for coaching and advice. You would also assume the more senior author position (i.e., the last author on a paper). If you are at the associate professor level, being first author can be an important factor for the appointment and tenure committee. This is also a time to collaborate in scholarship with people within your own field, outside your field, and within and outside your own institution. Adding breadth and depth to your experiences is important, which will help you develop a national reputation among your peers. By definition, the professor level implies you have attained recognition nationally, and certainly some of your colleagues will be able to write honest and detailed letters of recommendation for you as you strive to become a professor.

A last word about educational scholarship relates to funding. Whereas the funding of educational scholarship is ideal, it does not always free your time as expected. In my career, I received very little funding, although I did try. There just wasn't a lot of money available for education in those early days. The small amount of funding I did receive did *not* free my time for educational scholarship activities. As an example, I was funded for 15% to 20% of my time on a number of projects. In practice, I should have spent 15% to 20% less time in clinical activities, or one day a week. Logistically and in reality, there aren't faculty waiting in the wings to assume an extra day a week when one receives partial funding as I did. Basically, this formula for small grants never worked that way. In retrospect, negotiating small amounts of educational funding and determining how that factors into protected time is an area not well documented in the literature and needs to be addressed prospectively with the department chair. A word of warning is that being funded for a small percentage of time (5%–20%) on an innovative grant may not provide you with protected time and, in fact, might add yet another layer of responsibility on your already busy schedule.

ADVOCACY

Advocating for patients throughout your career should be part of the CE job description. Continuing this process as a mid-level CE in addition to becoming more vocal by interacting with the media, writing political representatives, and testifying at local, state, and national hearings around issues of importance to our patients are all activities within our abilities and reach. We can also rally our colleagues within our departments, at medical schools, and at national meetings on areas that impact our patients and all of us. There are so many instances where grassroots efforts to improve the health of people have made an impact, like mandatory wearing of bicycle helmets, crib safety for infants, and smoking cession, to name a few. Our voices as advocates might start out small, but adding others to our cause can get the attention of the people in power making critical decisions about health and safety.

MENTORING

This is the stage of one's career to be a mentor to junior-level CEs, within one's own institution and nationally. This group can also include residents, fellows, and medical students. As I was following the path of a CE, there was only one person locally (a PhD in my office) who was invested in education and could mentor me, so the rest of my mentors were from my national connections. That situation is different today, as there are many qualified mentors locally from which to choose. As junior faculty approach you as a potential mentor, having a discussion about why that person sought you out is important. Some might seek your mentorship on educational scholarship if you have a record of publishing. Others might admire your achievements based on gender and gravitate to you because of that. It's possible that a few faculty who are approximately the same genre as you might seek mentorship on keys to success at this stage. The initial goal should be to determine if there is a good fit between you and the mentee. That does not always happen, and I have suggested to medical students on a few occasions that I was not likely the best fit for them as a mentor.

Also, reading some of the literature on the characteristics of an effective mentor is certainly important. An understanding of the promotion process in one's institution is essential information for any mentor in order to be able to advise mentees appropriately. Suggesting promotion for a faculty member prematurely is not advisable, as a rejection can be viewed as lack of support from peers on one's performance. These issues can be discussed with the chair of the appointment, promotion, and tenure committee in the presence of the faculty member and you as mentor.

In some residency programs, residents choose mentors as safe counselors for ongoing evaluation of the resident's performance (i.e., milestones in the context of the competencies). The only word of warning here is not to take on more mentees than you can interact with comfortably, as some may need significant time. As part of your educator portfolio, document not only the faculty you mentor but their achievements regarding publications, awards, teaching accomplishments, and so on.

ADMINISTRATIVE RESPONSIBILITIES AND LEADERSHIP

As a mid-level CE, there are often opportunities to attain leadership positions in medical education. This could be the vice chair of education, a chair position in education at the medical school, chair positions nationally, and head of a task force around educational issues (e.g., developing a new curriculum), among other possibilities. By definition, CEs are not only vested in education but have furthered their career through advanced educational degrees, attaining educational expertise and theory through self-directed learning and, hopefully, some knowledge and skills about leadership (e.g., time management and how to run a meeting). Based on this experience, mid-level CEs are wonderful candidates to lead educational endeavors in the department, academic medical center, medical school, and nationally. Promotion and tenure committees generally value faculty attaining leadership positions, particularly when the CE documents how leading a committee or task force results in change and a tangible, usable product.

As a committee chair, it is critical that you learn how to delegate responsibilities and not assume all the work yourself. Again, this might be a good time of your career to reassess and revise your mission statement. As a mid-level CE, people will look to you to assume leadership roles. This can be an opportunity to further your teaching around educational principles and effect change in the educational arena. As chair of the Education Committee of the Academic Pediatric Association in the late 1980s, I was able to advocate for some issues that impacted the organization. An example was to encourage more educational abstracts and plenary sessions in the national meetings of the Academic Pediatric Association, the American Pediatric Society, and the Society for Pediatric Research, which was done in the early 1990s.

Lessons learned: There are many ways you can effect change in education through your teaching, educational scholarship, patient care, mentorship, and leadership. It was actually a challenge to get committee members to change their thinking about educational issues, and doing this top-down is not the best path to take. It happens more through a process I have labeled covert infiltration, in which you convert faculty through using evidence-based information and showing or modeling your passion and commitment.

4

The Senior Clinician Educator

By the time you reach the senior clinician educator (CE) level, it is likely that you have developed an area of expertise that is known not only locally but nationally, and that you have been promoted to professor on a non-tenured and, most often, a clinical track. That is not true of all faculty, as some remain at the associate professor level their entire careers. The age of attaining the professorial level of achievement is variable, and as stated previously, women are more likely to achieve this level a little later than men because of childbearing and taking the appropriate amount of time away from academics to tend to family. To avoid any criticism regarding gender here, men also take leave with the birth of a child, whether that be as a same-sex or opposite-sex couple. Data, however, have been limited to a woman conceiving and how that impacts achieving promotion and/or attainment of a PhD, with women achieving those milestones later than men in both medicine and science. For perhaps a myriad of reasons, like not being given leadership roles as they ascend the promotion ladder, not being afforded equal pay to men, and not being valued the same as men, women tend to leave and/or retire earlier from academic medicine than men.

RETIREMENT

As you become more senior, one of the most important professional critical events is when to consider retirement. So many factors impact this decision, like your financial status, clinical competency, downsizing to part-time status versus full retirement, job satisfaction, burnout, plans on what to do upon retiring, emotional well-being and general

DOI: 10.1201/9781003296270-4

health, spouse-related issues, and insurance coverage. Some variables have a major impact on the retirement process, like health, financial status, and financial obligations. It can be an emotional transition to leave a position that demanded total commitment to patient care, educational scholarship, leadership, mentorship, and teaching. For many, work can be all-consuming, leaving little time for hobbies and outside activities.

This being said, that commitment impacts what the retired CE might do upon exiting academic medicine. Leaving patients with whom you have worked for decades, in addition to separating from trainees and valued colleagues, can engender feelings of letting people down and abandoning the ship. These feelings can result in depression and concerns about self-worth if there is not some discussion and preplanning about what happens when this life cycle event takes place. A major concern is that, currently, many academic health centers provide little counseling for retirement, with two exceptions: (1) making certain one continues to receive health insurance from the academic health center, if available, or transition to Medicare; and (2) ensuring that one's finances are in order, assuming that faculty have participated in a profit-sharing plan throughout their careers.

Some of the questions that are not always addressed in academic health centers about pending retirement include the following:

1. When do you give notice if planning to retire?
2. If you plan to work only part-time, have you discussed that with the division chief and head of the department, and is this a viable option?
3. If you want to volunteer after retirement, what options are available in the academic health center and what credentials do you need (medical license, malpractice insurance)? Will the academic health center pay for these if you volunteer?
4. What are the options outside of medicine that would fit with your interests?
5. Are you eligible for and how do you apply for emeritus status?
6. How do you notify colleagues nationally that retirement is imminent?
7. Are there gender differences regarding the process?
8. Have you discussed plans for retirement with your spouse or significant other?

A story can illustrate issues around the retirement process. In 2000, I decided to leave full-time academic medicine because I had three grandchildren under the age of 5 that I was not seeing. Working 11- to 12-hour days and some weekends, I made a conscious decision to downsize and took a part-time job as the first head of faculty development at George

Washington University School of Medicine and Health Sciences. At 60 years of age and on top of my game academically, I was in no way ready for full retirement. The opportunity to move to a part-time job in an area that I loved was amazing and allowed me not only to see my grandchildren but to pick them up from nursery school and spend quality time with them. These are experiences that only come about once, and making a decision about how you prospectively view your priorities is important. Of course, I would not have made this move without the possibility of a part-time job offer, and I also had to discuss with my spouse the reality of a lower salary in making this major life adjustment. Some people thought I was crazy in doing this, and others considered it admirable. Looking back, I have absolutely no regrets financially, personally, or professionally. This decision-making was in sync with how I conducted the rest of my professional life, with a little of that bleeding into our personal lives (i.e., taking chances and grabbing opportunities that arose).

Thinking ahead and factoring in so many variables that are an integral part of one's career, there are many difficult decisions to be entertained and to be discussed with a significant other about retirement. Whether planning to downsize and continue part-time work or totally retiring, one should think ahead five years to make this process a well-thought-out and comprehensive one. Factors that come into play, as mentioned previously, include one's health and mental well-being, financial status regarding current and ongoing obligations, job satisfaction and question of burnout, competency in terms of caring for patients, and options available upon making this decision both within and outside the academic health center. CEs have a distinct advantage in both segueing to part-time work, as I did, or completely retiring. Having been an integral part of patient care, teaching, mentoring, educational scholarship, a community of learners locally and nationally, and leadership, there are potentially more options from which to choose if one considers staying connected to the academic health center. Discussing options with the division chief and the department chair is important. If finances are not a factor, one can choose to volunteer for some activities or negotiate small stipends for work.

When I assumed the part-time responsibility of faculty development at the medical school in 2000, the arrangement was a win-win for everyone. The school filled a gap that was essential to meeting the requirements of the Liaison Committee on Medical Education review in 2001, I was able to work in an area in which I had accumulated expertise, I was able to provide some support to faculty at George Washington University who had little to no exposure to educational theory and practice, and the medical school provided me with a reasonable salary and fringe benefits, which were necessary for me to make this move.

In addition to my responsibilities on The George Washington University main campus, I volunteered at Children's Hospital in the general pediatric ambulatory area, and my main duties were to observe trainees doing histories, physical exams, and counseling. This also filled a gap, as attending physicians at Children's were unable to observe trainees frequently, precluding their ability to assess milestones and competencies as required by the Accreditation Council for Graduate Medical Education. So, I fulfilled my objectives of staying connected to patient care and continuing my educational passion—teaching and educational scholarship.

Lessons learned at this stage of your career nearing retirement are many, and I have touched on them briefly. Finances tend to govern a lot of what we do and decisions we make. There are some known facts that need to be included in trying to assess future retirement needs. For example, CEs generally make less income than other specialists, and women make less than men at comparable positions. I realized that prospectively in my career and did some expert witness work in medical malpractice cases to enhance my income. That takes a toll, as the work has to occur in one's free time, cutting into family and leisure time. Based on some studies in the literature, it cannot be assumed that one's finances are in order at this late period. Making poor investments, not thinking about the future, and having major monetary obligations with children who are divorced or who themselves have had financial trouble are issues that are not always predictable. This can lead to underestimating what one needs to have a comfortable life, however that is defined, nearing retirement. Not having financial stability can determine how long one works, despite wanting to retire earlier in some instances. This can also be a factor in determining whether there is compensation for opportunities after full-time work.

It is also important to start thinking about what happens after retirement. The new you will be going from long workdays, and night and weekend calls, to lots of leisure time, unless, of course, you are writing a book! Exploring opportunities in staying connected to the academic health center should be planned well in advance, either as a volunteer or as a part-time faculty member. If that is not the plan, you need to determine what organizations in the community are an option. My wife and I deliver meals on wheels weekly, have been political activists by encouraging people to vote and have worked the election polls in November 2020, and volunteer to assist Holocaust survivors during festive occasions. I have also completed an application to volunteer at the

Library of Congress, put on hold during the COVID-19 pandemic. The other area that many retirees prioritize is travel, and planning this when one is healthy is ideal.

Some CEs lose their sense of identity and self-worth upon retirement and need activities to restore their ability to contribute to society. Depression is not unusual among retiring physicians. Segueing to a more leisurely lifestyle represents a goal for many, but some may need more structure. Priorities can, of course, change over time, but thinking about how you will fill some of your time is important. For some, it may be helping one's grandchildren with childcare or assisting with carpooling. For others, it may be ideal to start volunteering on a limited basis to see how this model fits with your needs. When I transitioned to part-time work, I also initially volunteered once a month to observe trainees perform history and physicals. Over time, what I had initially negotiated (i.e., one day a month) worked best for me, and I never saw the need to increase my time volunteering in the academic health center.

In summary, the retirement process is seldom addressed by academic health centers, and you need to be prospective about planning for this stage of your career, involving all the stakeholders. It is such an important extension of your career, and going into retirement in good health and being financially sound are factors that lead to being happy in those golden years.

MAKING AN IMPACT

The other important issue I observed as I attained senior status as a CE were requests from departments to facilitate workshops, many of them around teaching residents how to teach and improving their communication skills. Interesting that teaching residents how to teach was the first randomized controlled trial I conducted as a junior CE and published in 1982. As they say, what goes around comes around. When faculty would ask if I would conduct such workshops around adult learning, feedback, teaching a skill, and case-based teaching, I agreed to do that if (1) we looked at outcomes and developed an evaluation aspect of this effort, (2) we were willing to publish our results as educational scholarship, and (3) the contacting faculty could co-facilitate the workshops to ensure their continuation. It is evident where I am going with this model: provide teaching expertise to the department, engage a faculty member in this endeavor to educate that person and hopefully assure continuation of the workshops over time, collaborate on the curriculum as to logistics and how best to deliver the information to the residents, negotiate a rigorous evaluation to check the efficacy of the program, and finally, publish the results. I am proud to say that ob-gyn, anesthesiology, neurosurgery, and pediatrics all bought in to this model, and we published results in each instance. This is an example of how impactful one can be in the senior aspect of one's career. This is perhaps the most effective outcome of any project I have undertaken. We have co-facilitated our residents-as-teachers programs with key faculty from each of the departments, the programs have continued (with the exception of neurosurgery), we have published these results, and we have taught residents important educational skills.

Lessons learned: At the senior CE stage, you need to pay it forward and teach facilitative skills to others to ensure the continuation of programs. Helping more junior CEs publish in these areas is also important in your more senior position. It is most gratifying to see programs continue after you are no longer involved. This assures you that you have done your job and that your handoff was successful.

5

Tips for the Clinician Educator

Here are 35 tips clinician educators (CEs) were probably never taught in their medical school, their residency training, and perhaps, their academic career. They are divided into six categories: general (communication, reflection, and feedback), teaching, educational scholarship, patient care, administrative responsibilities and leadership, and personal life.

GENERAL: COMMUNICATION, REFLECTION, AND FEEDBACK

Tip 1: Recognize the Use of Silence in Interviewing and Teaching

My concern is that some of the evidence-based communication skills emphasized in my generation are giving way to technology. Research has been conducted on how much silence occurs once the physician asks the patient why he came in today. It is a matter of a few seconds and usually followed by a barrage of questions posed by the doctor. Unfortunately, this technique often precludes the patient from telling his story in full, meaning that not all the information that is critical gets reported. The interview can begin with a general question: "So, what brings you in today? How are things going?" Afterward, allow the patient to tell his story, with only occasional interruptions for clarification or probing comments made by the physician. Then one can fill in with the review of systems questions that complete the history. Remember that at least 80% to 90% of each diagnosis comes from the history and physical

DOI: 10.1201/9781003296270-5

exam, with additional information added by laboratory and imaging studies. There is a misconception that using a flurry of questions will shorten the interview process and be more efficient. Actually, allowing the patient the opportunity to tell his story, and then inquire about his main concerns and why those concern him, is a more effective way of getting information, with patient talk exceeding doctor talk.

In terms of teaching, silence allows the learner to think at higher cognitive levels if you are asking a lot of open-ended questions. Bloom's taxonomy, Miller's triangle, and Kirkpatrick's work assess levels of performance and cognition. I have observed that on inpatient rounds and in the ambulatory setting, faculty often use close-ended questions, requiring little or no thinking (recall) and one-word or minimal-word answers. However, when faculty employ more open-ended questions, greater depth of thinking and higher cognitive levels are required, and the trainee, in response, needs to think about the answer (unlike with close-ended questions). Again, allowing the learner to do most of the talking enables the teacher to diagnose that learner as to her previous experience with similar patients and overall knowledge. Silence can be difficult for the enthusiastic teacher, but remember how you are trying to effect maximum learning—and that doesn't happen with you doing most of the talking.

The lessons here are parallel for patients and learners: the teacher never has to be center stage but must be astutely able to facilitate great learning by activating learners, taking them to levels they were never sure they could achieve, and allowing patients to tell their stories. Silence allows learners to think cognitively at higher levels, similar to how expert clinicians problem-solve in the clinical setting. As for patients, giving them time to think about the problem they are coming in for can lead to a clinician's more complete assessment and approach to that problem. Silence is so unusual in either a teaching or patient care situation, probably because we need to practice it more and feel comfortable using it.

Tip 2: Be Reflective in Everything You Do

One of the books I read early during my mid-career was Donald Schon's *The Reflective Practitioner*, listed in the annotated bibliography. This treatise was life changing for me professionally, as it emphasized the importance of self-reflection in everything we do. Upon reading his book and hearing colleagues address this issue, I made reflection an integral part of what I did in my personal and professional life. Schon described the phenomena of reflection-in-action and reflection-on-action, while another group of educators identified reflection-for-action. To briefly summarize these processes, reflection is a valuable tool while seeing patients, teaching, and/or managing other academic responsibilities, like chairing a meeting. Reflection-in-action occurred in the moment or prospectively and enabled me to self-assess whatever I was doing, leading to change on some occasions.

As a teaching example of reflecting-in-action, when interacting with a student or resident and recognizing the learner was not understanding my teaching point, I considered another way to present that point. That same scenario can also occur with patient care. When during a history, you may not obtain the necessary information you need for the diagnosis and treatment, recognizing that problem prospectively can allow for reframing questions that may lead to better understanding by the patient and the information you are seeking.

Reflection-on-action occurs after the teaching episode and patient interaction, and is akin to a postmortem. You ask yourself how you think things went, what you thought of your relationship, and whether the patient or learner committed to change in their care or learning. Another important question is this: What could I have done differently that would have further enhanced the interaction?

Finally, reflection-for-action means thinking about how you would act in a similar situation in the future. This represents an adult learning principle: improving your behavior based on experience and self-reflection.

Story 1: One of the grand rounds topics I have presented numerous times is titled "How Do I Know I Am Teaching Effectively?" Each time I present this session, I am acutely aware of the faces in the audience, and I never stand behind the podium, which I perceive as a barrier between me and the audience. I use a roving microphone and teach by walking around the room as a way to engage people. I assess whether people are giving me eye contact, and this is how I use reflection-in-action. For this session, I have made decisions to reduce content based on how much time I have allowed for participants to comment on topics within the presentation. After each session, I reflect on how that session went and what I would do differently next time.

Story 2: One of my colleagues and I were facilitating a series of educational workshops for the neurosurgery residents. On one occasion, a workshop was delayed because the chief resident was in surgery, and the residents who were present were not happy because of the postponement of the workshop. I didn't address those feelings as

I started the workshop late, and my co-facilitator, recognizing this dissonance, called a time-out and intervened, acknowledging that we would modify the workshop so that we did not run overtime. The residents' agitation dissipated, and we went on with the workshop once this issue was confronted.

Lessons learned: I consider reflective practice to be one of the most important skills for CEs. Using this technique might require conscious behavior until it becomes an automatic and unconscious habit over time. I have found reflection to be the most important and powerful aspect of how I grew professionally. There is no need to read Schon's book to understand reflection, since there have been many review articles, including one by Plack and Greenberg in *Pediatrics* in 2005 and, more recently, one by Karen Mann, a longtime leader in medical education.

The example of the neurosurgery experience was reflection-in-action, and my colleague picked up on the residents' anxiety and intervened, diffusing the situation. This reflective practice can be in the moment and a powerful way to address what isn't going well, either with patients or trainees.

Tip 3: Be Open to Constructive Comments and Feedback by Peers

I have two stories that really say it all about this issue. For the first story, I was a second-year pediatric resident (1966) caring for a toddler who presented with diarrhea, vomiting, and excess salivation, and I did not immediately recognize that he had organophosphate poisoning. A peer of mine, prior to his residency, had served two years in the Army, where he learned about organophosphate poisoning, and he told me that he did not think this child had straightforward gastroenteritis. His astute observations and experience led to the correct diagnosis and treatment for this child.

The second story involved my caring for an infant with an infectious disease, about which I do not recall all the facts. I do remember, however, the head of infectious diseases at Columbus Children's (later to become dean of the Ohio State Medical School) critiquing my care of this patient in front of the entire team. I realized that he was correct in his assessment, and his comments inspired me to strive harder in paying attention to detail when dealing with patients. By chance, we passed each other in the hall the same day, and he stopped me to ask if I was all right following the interaction on rounds. I replied that I was embarrassed in letting the patient, myself, and the team down, in that order, and suggested that this was a great learning point for me.

Lessons learned: We obviously don't stop learning once we finish our training. There is much to learn from others, whether it be peers or those overseeing care we are providing. Our openness and willingness to receive constructive criticism and/or advice is very important for our professional growth. Whereas the culture of medicine in the past was not to ask for advice or help and doing so was seen as a sign of weakness, these two stories illustrate how working together can sometimes result in better outcomes and more accurate diagnoses for our patients. We should never be fearful, in a safe learning climate, to ask others for help or for a second opinion in any situation where we are unsure. Turning these situations into a learning experience should be the goal.

TEACHING

Tip 4: When It Comes to Curriculum Innovations and Educational Scholarship, It Is Important to Take Chances and Go Beyond Your Comfort Level in Being Creative

Part of having fun in one's career is accepting difficult educational challenges and being optimistic that most of these will end in success. Approaching educational scholarship with rigor, especially pertaining to the evaluation, is paramount to assuring success. That is why I have suggested starting with the evaluation of any proposed educational scholarship and working backward. The risk-taking part happens when there is no precedent for whatever educational scholarship you are contemplating. You can never be certain a de novo study will evolve into something statistically significant in the case of quantitative research or result in meaningful themes in qualitative research. When you are building on previous scholarship (Boyer's scholarship of integration or application), you do have some previous research on which to build, and hopefully, this new iteration will add to the literature.

Story 1: Looking in your own workplace for educational scholarship ideas and curriculum innovations, there are so many areas that need investigation, in addition to looking at variations on what has already been studied. As an example, one of my areas of focus has been studying residents, medical students, and fellows as teachers. My original randomized controlled study on residents as teachers was published in the early 1980s (Jewett et al. *J Med Educ.* 1982;57:361–366), and there have been a number of iterations since using techniques, such as standardized learners. More recently, with the advent of the flipped classroom in education and then medical education, I initiated a project with the then chief residents at Children's Hospital to study residents as teachers using the flipped classroom approach. This method calls for outside-the-classroom preparation (i.e., focused readings) before the workshops so that we can focus on performance in the actual workshop. This study was published in *Academic Medicine* (Chokshi et al. *Acad Med.* 2017;92:511–514) and really is a wonderful model for those who want to spend a day teaching residents how to teach. The resident participants enjoyed and valued the experience. This program, which is ongoing, emphasizes the attention to teaching and learning within the institution.

Lessons learned: Some CEs do educational scholarship along specific themes, and others, like me, look for gaps in the workplace that need to be addressed. I have always found that there are many areas the medical and educational communities have accepted as fact that have never been studied. The constant questioning of traditions, knowledge, and approaches to performance has been, for me, a key to how I developed my educational scholarship. Whereas there are themes to what I have studied over time, I have not focused on any particular area in depth with the exception of teaching residents, students, faculty, and fellows how to teach, and addressing communication skills. The bottom line is to be creative and take chances. That mantra has paid off in my career.

Story 2: In 1984, the Association of American Medical Colleges published a white paper titled "The General Professional Education of the Physician" or the GPEP Report. In that paper calling for reform in medical education, one section addressed the lecture as the major way faculty deliver information to trainees and colleagues. The paper provided evidence that this methodology does not change physician or trainee behavior, likely because it is not in sync with adult learning principles (i.e., activating learners, providing information that is contextual and related to patients the participants are seeing, providing or receiving timely feedback, and providing a vehicle for interaction).

Reading this report and hearing more about it while attending national and regional meetings of the Association of American Medical Colleges, I decided that the lecture series I included in my pediatric clerkship perhaps needed further analysis. I decided, based on the GPEP Report, that I was going to eliminate all lectures from the clerkship and advised the clerkship committee of my decision and the reasons for the major change. After hearing the evidence for eliminating the lectures, the committee voted in favor of the change. I informed the committee that I would train faculty currently giving lectures to the students to transform their lectures into case-based interactive sessions and extend the time of those sessions from 60 to 90 minutes. Medical students were very angry about this change, as they maintained that pediatrics had the best lecture series of all the clerkships. I tried to assure them that I wanted to convert these sessions into more learner-centered sessions as opposed to passive ones, making their learning more significant. Although I did not measure the impact of the change, when faculty, over time, sometimes reverted back to traditional lecturing, students voiced their concerns proactively and in their feedback. This case-based, interactive model has persisted for a number of decades in the clerkship. It is an excellent example of taking a chance by changing a program that was successful based on student feedback into one that was more learner-centered and evidence-based.

Story 3: So much educational scholarship evolves from information that has never been studied and has been taken for granted as truth. A case in point is a 1980s book on the *New York Times'* best-seller list called *The One-Minute Manager* by Blanchard and Johnson, which focused on reinforcing employees' good work by giving them timely feedback. A family practice group from Seattle published a variation of that model and called it the five-step micro-skills preceptor but did not study it. After reading the book and then the article, I decided that more adult learning principles needed to be incorporated into the model to make it more learner centered. Hence evolved the eight-step preceptor, which has been published and is currently used by faculty in academic centers across the US. What we added to the Seattle model were additional steps that were steeped in adult learning principles, namely, previous experiences with similar patients, future learning objectives based on the case, and the act of listening to the learner (meaning the learner is activated to develop a differential diagnosis and plan for the case). We published this model, I have facilitated workshops on this research, and it has been disseminated to many medical centers. This model is an example of case-based teaching that helps to organize the teacher and reminds her of the important steps to carry out when engaging a learner around patient care.

Lessons learned: Be innovative and take chances. With any new innovation, start with the end point in mind and figure out how to evaluate what you are doing. Of course, with any trailblazing innovation, there might be some failures, however you define that. When I think about this concept, I recall the *New York Times* best-selling book in the late 1990s, *Who Moved My Cheese?*, which cleverly described how a colony of mice had a choice to stay with the old, moldy cheese they had or venture out to see if they could find something better. The book illustrates the question: Are we happy with the status quo because it feels secure and does not have risk, or do we think about the fact that there may be better options? The model that seeks new knowledge and is more adventuresome, takes risks, and is unsure brought me more satisfaction in my career. My career has been based on the latter concept of looking for new ways to present medical education concepts and ideas. It also led to others recognizing my innovations; specifically, the pediatric clerkship I chaired was awarded the top teaching program in the country by the Academic Pediatric Association in 1995. An integral part of that award included the elimination of lectures in the clerkship, small-group bedside teaching rounds (interacting with attending subspecialty physicians and patients that students ordinarily wouldn't be exposed to on their rotations), home health visits, oral and written student group case presentations/teaching, a problem-solving exercise called instructor plays patient (Foley et al. *J Fam Pract.* 1978;6(5):1037–1040), and an inpatient and ambulatory experience for all students.

Tip 5: Think about Converting Your Top-Down Lectures into Interactive or Flipped Classroom Sessions

As mentioned previously, lecturing does not effect behavior change, whether it has to do with patient-oriented or educational content. That being said, it is incumbent upon CEs to develop interactive lecturing techniques by inserting questioning, patient interactions, and Hollywood movies to engage learners and illustrate themes from the lecture. This also can be accomplished by utilizing the flipped classroom or just-in-time teaching techniques, two evidence-based ways to activate learners. By having interaction with learners (even in a large venue, like grand rounds), the teacher is able to assess the level where some of the learners are, at the same time commanding the attention of those learners.

A story to illustrate this point involved expanding educational scholarship on previous work I had published. A colleague and I enlisted the chief residents at Children's to see if they would be interested in reviving a residents-as-teachers program I had started years earlier at Children's, except in this case, we would use the flipped classroom approach. The idea was to reduce the number of hours needed to teach this curriculum, enlisting second-year residents for one day for workshops that otherwise would have been much more time-consuming. Information that residents normally would have learned during the workshop was provided in readings before each workshop, and once we determined, through a short multiple-choice quiz, that the residents had mastered the knowledge, we were able to achieve higher levels of cognition and performance in the workshop itself using standardized learners (medical students). In essence, most of the workshop was devoted to residents practicing their skills. This work was published in *Academic Medicine* in 2017, and the program continues today.

Lessons learned: Lecturing, the mainstay of medical education for generations, has been proven to be an ineffective way to deliver information to participants, whether it be changing behavior or promoting lifelong learning. Based on this evidence, there have been many publications about how to transform top-down lecturing into interactive sessions with trainees. The literature informs us that participants' attention span is about 20 minutes, and it is during these interludes that one wants to engage the audience through questioning, showing video clips illustrating a point you have made, using a group interaction such as what happens in problem-based learning, introducing a case presentation, and using other similar techniques. Any way you can reengage the learner is appropriate here and will allow learners to make contextual connections, thereby remembering the information better over time. The flipped classroom and just-in-time teaching promote didactic learning outside the classroom and allow more hands-on practice and application in the workshop or classroom.

Tip 6: Incorporate Movies into Traditional Lectures as a Fun and Effective Way to Engage Learners

A transformational technique that has been part of every large group session I conduct—whether lectures, grand rounds, or large workshops—is the insertion of movie clips into the session from Hollywood and documentary films that contain content related to education. In fact, every time I watch a movie or documentary, I always ask myself if any segments might be valuable to incorporate into the teaching I do. Dr. Rich Sarkin, a valued colleague, friend, elite educator, and professional soulmate, introduced me to the use of films in educational sessions. Some of his early suggestions included clips from *Karate Kid 1*, *Ferris Bueller's Day Off*, *The Paper Chase*, and *Indecent Proposal*, among others. Along the way, I found *The Blue Angels* from the History Channel as a model to teach organizational and planning skills, *School of Rock* as a way to teach understanding of the principles of the topic and their application, *Dead Poets Society* to model what the teacher can do the first day of class to set learning objectives and expectations of how he wants learners to behave, and *The Doctor* and *Wit*, both of which illustrate giving bad news, among other movies. *Doctor in the House* is a wonderful example of the hierarchy that occurs on rounds, something we have unfortunately learned from the British model. These clips are all content-neutral (with the exception of the latter two, which are medical), and almost anything participants say is acceptable, as how they view the clips is all seen and interpreted through their own lenses. The clips are engaging, participants demonstrate very positive facial expressions during the movies, and each provides a talking point around something I had stated earlier in the session or workshop. It is important to use short clips (one to two minutes), as anything longer can detract from the focus of the session. I tend to use three to four clips per hour of the session, and I believe learners like my clips better than my talking. In my grand rounds presentations, I inject clips every 15 to 20 minutes, realizing that the attention span during a traditional lecture is about that time. This converts the session from one that is top-down to one that becomes interactive *and* requires participants to apply what I had stated earlier to the clip that I show, a higher-order function on Bloom's cognitive taxonomy.

Lessons learned: Video clips can be a wonderful complement to formal or scheduled teaching sessions you have developed. They can be powerful, content-neutral learning tools should you choose them carefully and decide what learning points they illustrate. As an example, the clip I use from *Dead Poets Society* is from the first day of class when Robin Williams sets the tone for how his poetry class will evolve. He basically has the students read the definition of *poetry* from a text and then tells them that poetry is how one interprets it, not what the text says. I like this clip because the teacher basically defines the content area and lays out his expectations that the students will come prepared for class by having read the poems ahead of time. His teaching is also creative, and participants in grand rounds can see that, perhaps, reflecting on their own teaching. There are so many examples out there of how teaching and learning are done effectively and ineffectively, and just as important, something in between and left to the lenses of the beholder. Two other examples of the first day of class are *The Paper Chase* and *Indecent Proposal*. In both clips, the teacher employs an interesting approach in setting the tone for future learning and the learning climate. Interestingly, law faculty have stated to me that *The Paper Chase* is exactly what happens the first day of many law classes.

Tip 7: There Are Ways You Can Create a Positive and Safe Learning Environment

One of the major characteristics of adult learning theory is that learners do best when their learning climate is safe and supportive. So, what are ways we can establish a safe learning climate? These include making certain that goals and objectives of a rotation are clear; roles, responsibilities, and expectations are enumerated at the beginning of each rotation; the responsible faculty members know learners by name; and learners are informed how their teachers want to be addressed (I have requested trainees call me Larrie, but they have suggested Dr. Larrie, less formal than Dr. Greenberg). Characteristics also include being open and truthful about what you do and don't know, using *I* statements ("I can remember when I was a student and how faculty and residents treated me"), making assessments transparent, showing a willingness to work with learners, and establishing a learning contract with learners regarding their expectations of the rotation, revisiting those periodically to determine how the learners are achieving what they set out to do.

Lessons learned: One of the most important and sometimes overlooked characteristics of effective teaching is establishing a safe and nurturing learning climate. Part of that climate involves the actual physical environment where one teaches. Sometimes we have control of that, and sometimes we don't. I have been assigned to teach as a visiting professor in rooms that are dark and have no windows. That is not an easy obstacle to overcome. A room may also not be appropriately heated or cooled, also affecting how learning occurs. What we do have some control over is how we engage learners from the outset and how we interact with them over time. If you have ever read Malcolm Gladwell's book *Blink*, you will appreciate the importance of first impressions and how those can be enduring. Starting out with a new group of students or residents and not making this moment memorable in a positive way can affect how these trainees subsequently perceive you and the rotation.

I love small talk as a way to engage trainees. Rich Sarkin, whom I referred to previously, told how he started his newborn nursery rotation with medical students. He would ask each to tell something significant about themselves and what they would be doing if they weren't in medical school. After all the students related their own stories, likely learning things about each other not previously known, he would then tell his story, following the format he suggested. I refer to this as a warm-up, a way to break the ice and get people to focus on each other as people and not just healthcare professionals. This humanistic approach also sets the learning climate for the rotation.

Tip 8: When You Are Asked a Question while Teaching, Avoid Answering the Question until the Learner Addresses It First

Although there is no specific story related to this tip, I do have extensive personal experience and want to relate it in context. When a trainee asks an interesting and provocative question on rounds or in the ambulatory setting, our job as faculty is to encourage learners to commit themselves before we relate our answers to challenging questions. I usually acknowledge that the question is an interesting one (if indeed it is; if it isn't, you can defer to others on the inpatient team and ask what they think rather than make constructive comments about the question). I then suggest to those raising the question that they have probably thought about the answer and ask if they could please share what they think. If the trainee asking the question really does not have an answer, then I ask other members of the team if they have ideas. This approach accomplishes a couple of things: (1) it activates learners on the team and gets them involved in the rounds, and (2) it allows me to diagnose the learners by discovering where they are in their experiences and knowledge about the topic. This principle of knowing where the learners are comes out of studies from one of the giants of medical education, David Irby. He suggested that as part of adult learning, it is important for the teacher to recognize learner levels before deciding what to teach. How would you know what to teach without knowing what your learners know and have experienced?

Lessons learned: Trainees always feel comfortable posing questions when the learning climate feels safe. (I address that earlier in my tips.) When the climate does not appear safe, learners may have some reluctance to pose or answer a question because of concerns about their limited knowledge and experiences or concerns that they are exposing inadequacies before an evaluator. Even when trainees do not know a patient's specific diagnosis, they should be able to describe, with specific questioning, what they think might be happening with the patient from a pathophysiologic point of view (i.e., whether it is inflammatory, genetic, cardiovascular, cancerous, etc.). Deferring questions to other team members is an excellent way to involve the entire team when provocative questions arise. When others have had their say, then faculty members offer their opinion. That allows them to reinforce those answers that are in sync with theirs and dissect those that aren't regarding how trainees approached the problem.

Tip 9: Assessing Where Learners Are in Their Knowledge and Experience Is Important in Determining What You Teach Them

In a classic 1978 article, Dr. David Irby, a leader in education and educational scholarship for decades, addressed how one diagnoses the learner before knowing what to teach that person. One of the most direct ways to do this is to ask the learner if she has ever seen a patient like this before. If the learner responds that she has seen a few patients like the one in question, the teacher might ask how she might help the learner around this particular patient. If the answer is that the learner has never seen a patient like this previously, then the teacher must decide what point or points would be the most poignant to teach in this situation. Please note that I say one or two teaching points, as more is not always better. Announcing that these are teaching points also distinguishes patient care from the educational aspect of the interaction. Concretely saying "I am now going to make a teaching point about this patient" is a great way to segue from patient care to teaching. This model also is an underlying principle in the flipped classroom, where the teacher provides some background information about the topic at hand, the learners read this information before interacting with the teacher at a later date, the teacher checks the learners' knowledge of the topic via a short multiple-choice quiz, and assuming the learners had mastered the information, the teacher proceeds to a more patient-applicable exercise, like a case-based discussion.

A story to illustrate this point occurred some 20 years ago when Rich Sarkin and I had a workshop accepted at a national pediatric meeting. We planned the entire workshop by email, and when we met at the conference, we went over our game plan. At the start of the workshop itself, we had prepared some questions for participants so we could assess what level they were at in their knowledge and experience. Upon hearing their responses, we looked at each other, called a time-out, and immediately realized that what we had prepared was too basic for this group. We decided that changing the overall goal of the workshop to a train-the-trainer session, in which we would be teaching them how to facilitate the same workshop or variation thereof at their home institutions, would be the best approach. Ground rules included stopping us at certain points and asking questions about the process, which allowed for a more in-depth understanding of what we were presenting. The workshop received rave reviews, which would probably not have been the case had we presented what we planned in advance.

Lessons learned: The time we have for teaching on the fly can be so short that making certain we know where the learner is in his knowledge and experience with a given patient is paramount. That information can be a starting point for our teaching, as I previously mentioned, with the eight-step preceptor. Simply asking if the trainee has ever seen a patient like this before is a great way to diagnose the learner and, subsequently, know what to teach. This model also incorporates feedback and challenges the learner to self-assess or reflect on how to improve his or her performance. Incorporating that principle with reflection-in-action can alert one to potentially change an approach if indeed the learners are at a different level than expected.

Tip 10: When Using Questioning Skills, Avoid Rhetorical Questions with Trainees, as These Kinds of Questions Make Assumptions about What Trainees Have Experienced or Know

An example of this kind of question is "I assume you all know how to give feedback, correct?" When the teacher asks this kind of question, individual learners feel intimidated, in that they might feel they are the only ones who don't know how to give feedback and are afraid to ask, as it exposes their inadequate knowledge. In reality, many others in the group may feel the same way but be reluctant to respond, based on how the teacher framed the question. Making assumptions about what trainees know or what kinds of patient experiences they have had is inappropriate and shortsighted.

Short story: I was working with a senior resident, and we were seeing a patient together who presented with enuresis. When I inquired how many patients the residents had seen with this diagnosis, he responded none. I was very surprised, as the likelihood of not seeing any children with this diagnosis by this time in his training was extremely low. Had I commented, "I assume you have seen a number of patients with this problem," the resident might have felt inadequate. So, we discussed what knowledge the resident had regarding the problem and then proceeded to make certain we had asked all the right questions concerning the diagnosis. The resident was grateful that I guided him through the important aspects of the history and physical exam, followed by how to counsel the parent and child.

Lessons learned: Residents' training can be variable, and as teachers, we shouldn't make any assumptions about what we think they should have experienced along the way. It is helpful to start an interaction with the resident regarding each patient with "How many patients have you seen with this diagnosis, and what have been your experiences along the way?"

Tip 11: Having Trainees Develop a Learning Contract at the Beginning of Any Rotation Is a Way to Activate Learners by Challenging Them with Defining What They Want to Learn in This Block of Time

Knowles proposed that faculty incorporate the use of a learning contract for learners as a way to convert them from passive to active participants, in the case of medicine, at the start of a rotation. The learners formulate what they project as their learning objectives, and they can revisit these mid-rotation to determine if they are succeeding in accomplishing what they set out to do. In reality, learners may have very specific objectives in mind that they want to experience because of their interests and possible career goals. On occasion, these objectives might not be realistic and, therefore, not likely achieved. That said, discussing this self-assessment process in a group a few weeks after trainees craft their contract can be a powerful tool for faculty to assess how learners are navigating the rotation. This process also reinforces a safe learning climate and conveys to learners that leadership cares. Listening to feedback from the group can be a powerful way to address gaps and dissect problems more prospectively as opposed to waiting until the rotation is over.

Tip 12: Perfecting How You Frame and Give Feedback Can Make It a Humanistic Habit

Receiving timely, constructive, and reinforcing feedback is one of the major deficits that medical students and residents report in their training. Faculty who have not been trained to give feedback perceive that it is a timely process and have not always adopted a model that works for them. My longtime colleague, Jim Blatt, Professor of Medicine at George Washington University, has developed an acrostic based on Lawrence Weed's model for recording in the medical record: SOAP. This model is easily memorized, and the components are understandable. The *S* is "subjective" and translates into "How did you think things went?" This is an adult learning theory principle in having the learner self-assess or reflect on the interaction, thereby activating the learner and allowing the teacher to identify where the learner is. The usual response is "I think I did okay." That is followed by something like "Tell me what you think you did well and what can you improve upon." The *O* stands for "objective", and the CE tells the learner what she observed in the observation. "I noted that you did not probe the patient about her pain and why she seemed concerned about that." The *A* is the "assessment" of the observer on the overall performance of the trainee. "Basically, you have conducted the interview very well and you only have to fine-tune a couple of areas that we discussed. Your interpersonal skills were engaging for the patient and will be important to replicate." The *P* represents the "plan" for the future, again activating the learner to think about what she can do the next iteration to make this interaction even better. In general, it is quite rare in my experience over almost 50 years in the field that there isn't something constructive to offer. On that rare occasion, reinforcing what the trainee did well is the best way to provide this feedback.

Another important caveat about feedback is that we should not brand it as negative or positive. I often hear faculty characterize feedback in those terms. This has implications for the learner, especially when some of the feedback is constructive or corrective (Hewson and Little, *J Gen Int Med*, 1998). In fact, no matter what we do in any aspect of our lives, we all have room for improvement, and we should be labeling this as constructive or corrective feedback. Often overlooked by faculty is giving reinforcing feedback or telling the learner what they have done well. By emphasizing what the learner has done well, they are more likely to continue that aspect of their performance.

Lessons learned: Having a framework on how to give feedback in a timely, effective, and efficient way is important, and the SOAP format is easily memorized and applicable in the clinical situation. Counter to faculty perceptions, giving feedback to trainees after each patient encounter takes very little time and promotes professional growth of the learner within the competencies and milestones. Documenting oral feedback on a clinical encounter card can be used for summative feedback on any rotation (Ottolini et al. *Teach Learn Med.* 2010;22:97–101). Making this feedback model a humanistic habit and, eventually, an unconscious part of how you teach will benefit your trainees.

Tip 13: Utilize the Model of Activated Demonstration when You Show a Trainee a Physical Diagnosis or Interviewing Skill

There will be many opportunities over the course of your career to demonstrate a skill to residents and medical students. So often, faculty have a trainee enter the room with them, and do not activate the learner as they are observing that demonstration. ("Come with me into the room and watch me interact with the patient.") This activation represents a principle in adult learning (i.e., andragogy) and makes the learning so much more contextual and participatory. In this technique, the faculty and trainee discuss the skill that will be the focus of the demonstration and what the trainee's role will be while observing that skill. For example, the resident might have asked for your assistance in dealing with an angry patient. Her concern was that no matter how much she tried to diffuse the situation, the patient did not seem to be amenable to a pleasant interaction. You suggest to the trainee to watch how you first engage the patient, like what words you use and the body language you and the patient assume during the encounter. You also encourage the trainee to assess what is different about your interaction and her interaction with the patient. Once you exit the room, set aside a short time to debrief what transpired and what the trainee observed and learned.

Lessons learned: Applying adult learning principles to whatever teaching and learning situations you are in will help you build some humanistic habits that become part of your being, going from a consciously incompetent situation to one of unconscious and competent seen in more seasoned physicians. Activated demonstration is one of those areas where you can activate a learner to ensure maximum learning in situations where faculty demonstrate skills to trainees. The latter are transformed from a passive observer to one who is actively engaged, making effective and transformative learning likely.

Tip 14: First Impressions Are So Important, and Starting an Interaction with an Individual or a Group that Is not from the Heart, Engaging, and Learner-Centered Can Be Very Difficult to Undo

I referred earlier to Malcolm Gladwell's book *Blink* as an example of this. Being engaging and enthusiastic about new interactions is not exactly easy, especially when they are so repetitive, like having to engage trainees every few weeks or monthly as they start a new rotation with you. You have to approach this effort as if it were the first time you have done it, showing enthusiasm and the desire to partner with the trainees.

Story: As a longtime clerkship director, among my other responsibilities, I always engaged the students the first day of the rotation and challenged them with the statement, "If this is not the best educational experience in medical school, I want your feedback to tell me why." We also had initial conversations about their experiences in their previous clerkship rotations and addressed with them how pediatrics might be different. I tried to set the tone on day one that this was going to be hard work but fun and meaningful. I believe that this approach was a winning one, as our clerkship was always rated the best at George Washington University based on the dean's office's feedback. Parenthetically, I know some clerkships may have information available mostly online, in sync with how current trainees are used to learning information. This precludes your ability to engage the group and demonstrate your passion and ability to challenge the group on day one, setting the learning climate for the rotation.

Tip 15: When You See a Problem with a Trainee that Involves His/Her/Their Performance Being Below Standards, Discuss the Issue with the Trainee and Record that in the Individual's Record

There are times when one encounters behaviors of trainees that are outside the norms of the Accreditation Council for Graduate Medical Education competencies or milestones and need to be discussed with the trainee. In my experiences, many of these incidents fall into five categories: (1) nonprofessional behavior; (2) the possibility of learning disabilities not previously recognized; (3) the presence of emotional distress, illness, or substance abuse; (4) problems with organizational skills; and 5) psychosocial issues. Any of these categories can result in inadequate performance by the trainee, a red flag for faculty who oversee medical student, resident, and fellow performance. Once you see performance that is below expectations, meet with the trainee and voice your concern, being objective. Here's an example: "Faculty have informed me that you have been late to rounds and are often not prepared with information about your patients." If the trainee volunteers information that would address the subpar behavior, acknowledge that these kinds of issues need to be conveyed to the appropriate leadership position prospectively so everyone can work together to overcome the problem.

Depending on the root cause of the situation, counseling could lead the trainee down the correct path. As an example, if the problem is substance abuse, the appropriate parties need to be notified, and the individual needs to take a leave of absence and seek counseling or treatment. It is important that this information becomes an official part of the trainee's record according to the Accreditation Council for Graduate Medical Education competencies.

One of my concerns is that I have observed the situation where the trainee performs below standards in a specific area, with no past history of any similar reports. In some instances, faculty are reluctant to report that incident to the appropriate training program director, considering it an isolated occurrence. I would maintain that when we see substandard performance in a trainee, we meet with that trainee to determine the etiology and underlying explanation for the performance. Often, that meeting helps to define what has happened, and the trainee can work on his performance over a given time to make certain the problem is resolved. If the problem is not resolved over that time, the training program director will need to counsel the trainee and determine the viability of continuing in the program. We inform the trainee we are reporting the issue and that if indeed it is an aberrant incident, it will not likely remain in the record or be reported to those seeking information about the trainee. I can say that over the years, I have discovered previously unknown problems, such as learning disabilities, substance abuse, emotional distress over family and other issues, and illness-related reasons, for substandard performance.

Story 1: A number of years ago, one of the faculty reported that a third-year medical student did not seem organized on rounds and was having difficulty with assimilating information on his patients. He was otherwise always on time, engaged, and professionally appropriate. I agreed to observe his behavior on rounds and found the reported behavior to be true. When I counseled him, I told him our concerns, and he expressed frustration in not being able to assimilate information, resulting in good decision-making. He stated he was staying up until early morning hours reading about his patients and was exhausted. I asked to see his pediatric textbook, and the section he showed me revealed that *every* line on the few pages I examined was underlined. I immediately wondered about a learning disability and reported my discussion with him to the dean of students, who recommended developmental testing. It is amazing that this student reached this point without it ever being an issue. It's the difference between book learning and taking care of patients.

Story 2: I recently worked with a resident on a project to submit to a journal. I asked the resident to work backward from the time he expected the paper to be finished and establish doable timelines leading up to completion. I emphasized that priorities were his personal and professional life, then this project. I also recommended that he delegate any part of the paper to me if that was helpful and that contacting me monthly would be fine. This individual would be the lead author, assuming he adhered to the ground rules on which we mutually agreed. Unfortunately, the resident was unable to meet the set requirements. After not hearing from him for ten weeks despite a number of messages asking for his update on the project, I sent an email that established closure to our collaboration, providing feedback on what the resident did well and what was not done as mutually agreed upon. Not hearing back after sending the email, I contacted the training program director and stated that this was not only disrespectful but nonprofessional behavior and should appear as such in his record. The pushback was that this seemed to be an isolated incident for this resident, and my response was that it did not preclude it being included in his record as an objective observation (i.e., nonprofessional behavior). In counseling, I always say to a trainee that if this specific performance is an aberration, that is great. If it is part of a pattern, the trainee needs to address it to avoid future problems perhaps impacting patients, peers, and himself.

EDUCATIONAL SCHOLARSHIP

Tip 16: When You Develop a New Curricular Innovation, It Is Best to Start with the End in Mind and Determine How to Best Assess the Effectiveness of the Program

My anecdotal experience is that junior faculty (and sometimes more senior faculty) develop innovative educational programs with little attention to the best way to evaluate them. When you don't have a rigorous evaluation, you cannot share your innovations with peers through journal publications and national presentations. Without an appropriate evaluation to assess the program effectiveness, peers cannot determine if the program is evidence-based and adaptable in their setting. When you start to conceptualize a new curriculum, laying out the goals and objectives is the first order of business, followed by the methodology of how you will address those goals and objectives. Finally, and most importantly, how will you evaluate what you have set out to do in a rigorous manner? I have maintained that every new curricular innovation is worthy of publication if one adheres to these principles.

Story: Early in my career when I was clerkship director, I had an epiphany that I wanted to send medical students on pediatrics out to patients' homes accompanying health professionals who were already scheduled for those visits. The students were assigned a specific half day to meet at an agreed-upon point with a healthcare professional, usually at a metro stop and occasionally linking by car. They then traveled to a patient's home, with the patient or parent having been advised in advance of the student's presence. Once entering a home, the medical student was required to assess the patient's status, assess the physical aspects of the home in the context of the child's illness, assess the health professional's responsibility (usually a nurse, a social worker, or a physical therapist), and do a final assessment of the visit. The students were required to write a narrative reflection on the visit, addressing the earlier points at a minimum. They had a deadline for submitting the narrative. I read all their narratives, making comments on the issues included and not included that seemed pertinent; I returned the narratives and graded them pass or fail. We then had an hour-long review session to discuss some of their experiences, and I had specific students report on their visit to illustrate important points in front of the entire group.

Here's the rub. This curricular innovation occurred early in my career as a CE. Although I had researched the literature on home visits by medical students (which was very limited at the time) and discovered that this program was innovative and a complementary part of the students' experiences on pediatrics, I was not informed enough about qualitative research, which, in retrospect, was the best way to evaluate this program. The reflective sessions with students relating their experiences were so interesting and powerful that I often learned nuances about patients and families that I didn't know existed. Had I known how to do qualitative scholarship at the time, I would have been able to enlist another faculty member with expertise in that methodology, and we could have collaborated on this endeavor, extracting common themes that resonated from student experiences. Although I published the results of the study, it would have been a stronger publication had I utilized qualitative methodology. Parenthetically, only educational journals accepted qualitative research at the time.

Again, the lesson learned here is to decide how to measure what you are studying before beginning the study. It was not until later in my career, with help from more expert faculty, that I engaged in qualitative research. In fact, one of the things I did well in my career was enlist talented colleagues in my research—some fellow pediatricians, others that were nonphysicians with educational backgrounds, and some from other disciplines I would label value-added to the project. Some of them brought context expertise, but most were experienced in methodology and design. As I gained experience, at the start of an idea, I always asked myself about the key players who needed to be a part of the project to make it not just successful but beyond that. Sometimes these key collaborators are within your division or department. Others may be within the university, and the rest may be found nationally, such as physicians, educational researchers, or occasionally, experts outside of medicine.

Tip 17: When Doing Collaborative Educational Scholarship, It Is Very Important to Determine Early in the Process the Responsibilities, Timelines, and Order of Authors on Abstracts and Papers Submitted

Understanding the workings and logistics of academic medicine is critical in undertaking educational scholarship. If the innovation on which you are collaborating is your concept and idea, it would make sense that you would be the principal investigator and first author on the study. This can be a formidable task for a junior faculty member learning all the nuances of a new job. Although there are faculty at this level who are great at time management and delegating responsibilities to others, I would advise that you not assume this role until you have more experience under your belt, which can vary depending on the individual.

Therefore, when starting out in educational scholarship, the best alternative may be to be a vibrant member of the team but not the principal investigator. The team involved in the study would negotiate roles and content areas on which they would work, with a timeline agreed upon by all. My view of timelines is to start with when the group thinks the actual paper will be ready for publication and work backward, using realistic deadlines. Among the roles inherent in doing educational scholarship are recruiting subjects, preparing informed consent (if people are involved), conceptualizing the research design and evaluation, submitting a proposal to the institutional review board, and considering how the study content fits with specific journals and national organizations or meetings.

At the early stage of project development, the author order is important to establish with all parties in agreement. If the collaborators are all junior, my suggestion is that the principal investigator (usually the one who takes overall responsibility) be the first author on the major paper that evolves from the educational scholarship. The promotion and tenure committee, when evaluating faculty worthiness of promotion to the next academic level, places major emphasis on the order of authors on papers, abstracts, and book chapters or books. Being first author has significance, and this should not be underestimated. If another team member is senior, that individual usually has her name last in the order of authors. A mid-level colleague might also need first authorship; based on his level of involvement, that can be negotiated with the team.

On some occasions, there might be two or more papers from a study, and first authorship can be rotated among the authors—again, assuming the lead author does the major part of the work for that submission. There are also possibilities that the study results in a paper, **and** a variation can be submitted to another journal, like MedEd-PORTAL, perhaps describing the study in detail to enable faculty to duplicate and apply it at their own institution. I have often submitted abstracts to both pediatric and medical education organizations, listing acceptances with one acknowledgment on my CV. For example, if the abstract is accepted in three different meetings, it is listed once. The reason for multiple submissions is that these groups have different audiences and input from each is valuable. Again, a single study can result in a number of publications, enabling coauthors to share in first authorship.

Lessons learned: Doing collaborative studies or scholarship is a very complex task, with a variety of barriers and roadblocks: authorship order, delegation of responsibilities, timelines (which should be somewhat flexible), and group work. It is important to consider some of these issues before going down this path, even when the most senior member of the team doesn't address them. It is not unusual for someone in the study not to keep to timelines or complete responsibilities as agreed. That makes for difficult interactions and resentment among team members, and certainly, the most senior member of the team should take the lead here (if they are not the irresponsible one) to help resolve this issue. If there is no mid-level or senior-level person, perhaps the group should ask the director of medical education or someone involved in research or educational scholarship for advice and to, perhaps, intervene under extreme circumstances. In essence, when the ground rules are clear from the beginning, there is less chance of problems occurring later on.

Unfortunately, I have a story about one study with a senior medical student that was never completed. We established ground rules from the start, with her taking the lead and setting timelines. I was able to provide her with important information in the beginning, which I assumed would make the task easier for her. Over time, I observed some major communication issues with her, and she did not respond to my emails in a timely fashion. The crux of the problem was her not adhering to timelines that *she* had established and that we had agreed upon from the start, and not informing me why. In essence, I dismissed her from the study with careful written and oral documentation, also informing the dean of students at the school. This was most uncomfortable for her and me, but the solution chosen was the only way to resolve an ongoing problem. She subsequently related a series of personal and family problems that she was experiencing over time, and I was empathetic. However, she was remiss in not relating these issues to me prospectively and not responding to my communications to her. I hope this was a learning experience for her, and I related that if she approached similar problems the same way during her residency or in practice, she would be putting herself, her patients, and her career in jeopardy.

Tip 18: Recruiting Medical Students and Residents to Partner with You in Your Educational Scholarship Is a Win-Win Outcome

As I approached the end of my mid-career as a CE and moved into my senior level, I actively sought out senior medical students enrolled in the elective on teaching medical students how to teach to collaborate with me on educational scholarship. There were also pediatric residents with whom I interacted who were either required to do a research project or were chief residents that showed an interest in medical education scholarship. In every instance in which I worked with a trainee, I taught them the importance of negotiating authorship; doing this work in snippets and not waiting for large blocks of time to become available; setting timelines compatible with one's daily routine, starting from when the educational scholarship project is to finish and working backward until the present; dividing responsibilities; thinking about journals that would be potentially receptive to this kind of research; keeping in contact periodically for updates on the project; using the opportunity to submit abstracts to different organizations with different audiences (e.g., Association of American Medical Colleges, either national or regional meetings, specialty-specific); and being available for mentorship at any time.

I found trainees perhaps lacking in research experience, but they always surprised me with creative ideas and suggestions, prospectively. The fact that they were willing to share informs me that they felt that the environment was trusting and that I was receptive to listening.

The many educational scholarship projects on which I collaborated with trainees almost always resulted in abstract submissions and presentations to a number of national organizations, and on occasion, there was more than one paper from the research. As noted earlier, first authorship can change when there are multiple submissions, such as abstracts and manuscripts. A few trainees assumed full responsibility for the statistics and methodology; others did some of this work, and I and/or the coauthors did the rest.

Lessons learned: Collaborating with trainees has been a mutually rewarding experience and has resulted in publications most of the time. Medical students and residents bring fascinating ideas to projects, have a great work ethic, and are enjoyable to work with. In return, I can teach them methodological design, evaluation, journal selection, time management, and coaching for presentations nationally. What is most gratifying is seeing our work published and having the trainees bask in this achievement. Over 85% of work started with trainees resulted in publication, with both papers and abstracts. Unfortunately, losing track of trainees once they leave the institution is the norm. From that perspective, it is difficult to know how much of an impact I have had on my fellow collaborators. I can only optimistically hope they have learned through these experiences and applied some of the principles to their future endeavors. I do know that some have continued to publish papers, and occasionally, I have interacted by email with some.

Tip 19: Don't Look for Protected Time to Do Your Educational Scholarship

I worry that junior CEs look for protected time to do unfunded research, and it is not there. Even when I had small funded grants that would pay 10% to 15% of my time, there was no way I could use that as protected time to do my educational scholarship. Trying to balance personal and professional life also factors in here, so my advice is to get a plan each time you conduct a study. Unlike basic science research in the laboratory, one can do educational scholarship in allotted time frames—an hour here, a half hour there. Think about the time you want to devote to family and other outside interests, and what times each week you are going to devote to your study or paper. This can be small aliquots of time to write specific sections of the paper (introduction or methodology) or to devote to the study itself, like the statistical assessment. Making educational scholarship a priority, although not necessarily a top priority, will help you finish your study and write your paper. Being organized like this will bode you well for completing educational scholarship in the future as you build your career.

I have seen many CEs who have problems balancing their educational scholarship and other responsibilities. I am not certain they comprehend the concept of devoting small amounts of time to a project and adhering to whatever schedule they set for this. Timelines can be moved when unanticipated events occur. Either the educational scholarship is a priority in context or not. For some, educational scholarship will not be an integral part of their mission statement, and they will try to excel in other areas of the mission.

Lessons learned: Despite lacking formal training in research methodology and statistics, I was determined to make educational scholarship a significant part of my career. I had to do this work as part of my time away from the institution (nights and weekends) but was able to share the work with co-collaborators and fit this into my schedule without a negative impact on my family. When you have passion, you make things work, and this is how CEs develop a portfolio of excellence. By the way, I have always found publishing my work illuminating, and I am proud it has hopefully enhanced the field.

Tip 20: You Can Make a Poster Session at Meetings More Educationally Meaningful and Interactive

Poster sessions on educational scholarship are an integral part of national meetings and often fill large convention center halls with unending aisles of posters accepted for presentation. Anecdotally, I most often see junior faculty and trainees manning the posters, and when I stop briefly to read the essence of the study, most study authors do not reach out and ask if they can help sort through details for me. Because most posters are filled with lots of numbers and detail, and there are so many available to view, one has to question why people might stop to see my poster.

Having had numerous poster presentations, I have developed an approach that makes the session more engaging. When I see participants stopping ever so briefly to gaze at my poster, I immediately make eye contact and offer to summarize the essence of the study for them. I have never had a person walk away when I ask this, and thus, I have an immediate audience to whom I can explain my work or study. It often happens that others passing the poster, seeing a few people talking, will also stop and listen to my brief presentation. This proactive approach engenders many more discussions about the study and precludes participants from having to read through all the information on the poster. This technique has resulted in an occasional collaboration and newfound ideas based on the interactions.

Tip 21: Interact with Journal Editors on Your Educational Scholarship Submissions

Two stories: In the early 2000s, a recently retired editor from a prestigious educational journal was in the Washington, DC, area, and I was able to recruit her to conduct some faculty development workshops at George Washington University on preparing and submitting papers to journals. One of the things that has stayed with me all these years was her suggestion to send an email to journal editors briefly describing your intended submission to assess if that journal is the best fit for your study. In fact, I have sent out abstracts to two to three journals simultaneously and waited for replies. On one occasion, two journals actively solicited my paper, and I was able to choose which journal to submit to. The email to the journal(s) should include an abstract of the paper for the editor's perusal. There is a lot of competition among journals to publish great scholarship, and *some* editors have replied to me over the years based on my emails to them. None has committed beyond stating that the content seemed in line with the journal mission and goals, and to send it on. A few have suggested that a proposed article does not seem to be appropriate for the journal or that a manuscript would have to include certain specifics in order to be reviewed. This information can be helpful in deciding where to send an article and can save months' time by not sending to a journal whose editor is reluctant about the appropriateness of the article for that journal. Lastly, most journals indicate that they cannot comment without seeing the paper first, so you are back to square one on deciding where to submit.

A second story happened with a well-known editor who had rejected a paper that addressed giving bad news in a one-day workshop for seven critical care fellows in our pediatric program. Our fellowship program in critical care had eight fellows, with one being the lead author on the study. Retrospectively, we should have used qualitative methodology for the assessment; however, the authors used a quantitative approach to assess the effectiveness of the workshop. Few pediatric journals were accepting papers with qualitative research in those days (the late 1990s), a factor that led us away from that methodology. Understanding that traditional statistics are not valid with such a small number of study participants, we downplayed statistics in the paper but mentioned that the trend was encouraging for the success of the intervention (Vaidya et al. *Arch Pediatr Adolesc Med*. 1999;153:419–422). The reviewers' comments were quite complimentary for the methodology, as this was a unique way to teach giving bad news—that is, a one-day approach using interactions with one set of standardized parents in the morning followed by feedback on the content and communication skills. In the afternoon, the fellows engaged another set of standardized parents with a different but similar case scenario to determine if they learned and applied content and communication skills from the morning session. However, the paper was rejected because of the small sample size and statistics that were not a value-add for the paper. Based on very positive reviews and the fact that we reported data on all the fellows that comprised the fellowship at Children's, I contested the rejection and suggested that the paper be reviewed by one more person before a final decision was made. The editor listened to my concerns and recruited another reviewer, and the paper was eventually published and has been cited more than 110 times.

One more example is that we recently had a paper rejected on a topic not at all well published and of extreme importance to trainees and faculty. The paper needed a lot of logistic changes to adhere to the journal's guidelines, and the editor basically encouraged us to resubmit an edited paper after having rejected the paper on two occasions. He obviously wanted to publish the paper but only after we made significant edits, which we did. The paper was recently published. Note that incorporating revisions suggested by a journal does not guarantee publication of the paper.

Third story is one I have told many times. In 2005, I wrote the editor of *Pediatrics*, the most-read journal in our field, to inform him that there was no evidence in pediatrics of any studies or articles on the important subject of reflection. I said that my coauthor and I had written a review article on the topic, and he encouraged that we submit the article. It never made it out of the editor's office, and we received an acceptance within a week. This scenario doesn't happen often, but emailing editors with suggestions sometimes works.

Lessons learned: I know that my experiences in this area cannot be generalized to all situations, but a carefully worded email or abstract to a few journals in parallel fashion asking if your paper might be suitable for the journals in question is a reasonable approach. On one occasion, I had two replies from interested editors, and I chose Journal A over Journal B, eventually replying to the editor of Journal B that the paper was accepted by another journal and thanking him/her. If Journal A rejects the paper, then one can submit to Journal B.

The second lesson is humbly questioning an editor when reviewer responses are positive, and/or both the journal and you know the importance of publishing the subject matter can promote second thoughts for the editor in having you resubmit the article after edits following a rejection. Your persistence is critical when the majority of the reviewers' comments are glowing but the paper is rejected by the editor for whatever reasons. Know that you have some power, although limited.

Tip 22: With Few Exceptions, There Is Almost Always a Journal that Will Accept Your Educational Scholarship, Unless Your Study Has a Fatal Flaw or Your Commentary Does not Add Value to the Current Literature

Of course, perusing a journal's table of contents to see what it publishes and its impact value is a good start to determine to which journals to submit your study or commentary. I am reminded that Dr. Seuss had his original submission to publishers rejected over 30 times. Based on that, it's important to listen to the feedback you have received from editors who have rejected your paper and incorporate comments that relate to the methodology and results. That said, I have received feedback that would have required a total rewrite of the paper in addition to changing the methodology. In those situations, I confer with my coauthors on next steps. It is an exception where I have had to change my total approach toward the study. Look for bibliographies that list medical education journals or journals that accept educational scholarship. Some are from North America and some from the continent. There are numerous journals outside North America that have worldwide readership but also a stringent peer review process. There are other recognized journals with a slant; for example, *The American Medical Student Research Journal* is a great fit if you are publishing with medical students as first authors. I have three to four publications in that journal, and in each instance, the student is the first author.

Lessons learned: Unless an editor relates to you that your paper has a fatal flaw in the methodology, there are journals that will accept your paper. It might take a few iterations to get the paper published; just stick with it. When I have a collaborator, I think about all the work and time that went into creating the study and writing the paper, and that is what spurs me on. I have worked with colleagues who react negatively to rejections and basically give up publishing the paper.

I guess I am suggesting that if the commitment and passion is there, you will find a publisher. Journal rejections are not rejections of you; the rejections are multivariable and can reflect how the study fits with the journal content and standards, the way your methodology is viewed, and the depth of your evaluation. I have performed a few observational studies that have not been received well by some journals but have still been published.

PATIENT CARE

Tip 23: Enhance Your Patient Communication Skills by Asking the Right Questions

An overlooked body of research on patient care and interviewing skills is that of Dr. Barbara Korsch, who was a pioneer in studying gaps in doctor-patient communication in the 1960s and 1970s. Her seminal research on studying pediatric residents' communication skills revealed major omissions in their identification of **what** the patient's or parent's main concern was (which was sometimes quite different than the chief complaint) and in their probing of **why** the patient was concerned. When surveying parents in exit interviews after an ambulatory visit, she found that residents asked these questions only 25% of the time. Not really knowing or understanding what concerned the patient and why that concerned him or her can result in continued anxiety for the patient, lack of trust in the relationship with the doctor, and possible nonadherence to medical advice. For the asking physician, not understanding what the patient's major concerns are and why can lead to missed information and unnecessary return visits. Based on her research, asking these questions at each encounter, which literally takes seconds, strengthens the doctor-patient relationship and can increase the relationship with the physician, who would be more likely to be perceived as caring. We need to use these questions in our own practices and then teach them to trainees; they are an important tool for trainees to have in their patient encounters.

A story to illustrate this point occurred a number of years ago during the latter part of my career when a junior resident presented an 11-year-old preadolescent to me with a chief complaint of a tender lump and enlargement of one breast. I already knew the diagnosis before entering the room based on my experience with previous patients like this, an educational term known as pattern recognition. I asked the resident what the main concerns were of the mother, and he stated she just wanted her child checked out. I instructed the resident to watch how I would question the patient or parent (a technique called activated demonstration: *Tip 13*) and elucidated the main worry and why that worried both of them, especially the mother. I entered the room and introduced myself as the resident's supervising physician. I asked permission to examine the patient and corroborated the fact that she had a tender, moveable, quarter-sized mass under the areola of her left breast and mild gynecomastia, compatible with the onset of puberty. I then proceeded to ask the patient if she had any concerns. Typical of many preadolescents, she did not express any. I then deferred my attention to the mother and asked if she had any major concerns about the chief complaint and physical findings. She denied any. Realizing I wasn't likely to get an answer through my usual questioning, I then asked her, "What do you think about when you hear about a mass in someone's breast?" She quickly replied, "breast cancer," illustrating the importance of elucidating the main concern and reason for that concern. In the counseling, I emphasized that her daughter did not have breast cancer, and that was 100% certain. I then went on to explain the issue about the onset of puberty, and I believe that the patient and her mother exited the interview relieved to hear my comments. The other value-added point that emerged was that in the reflective discussion with the resident after the interview, he recounted the questioning he observed during my interview and how the parent responded to these questions. Here again is an example of contextual teaching around the care of a patient.

So, the lesson learned here is obvious: Incorporating these two questions into your interviewing techniques is critical to determine the patient's main concern and why that concerns her, the end result being increased patient satisfaction and adherence to medical advice, and a better physician understanding of the patient's problem.

A second story is how one promotes activation of the patient in the counseling process. I have learned over the years that just telling the patient to do something doesn't always result in their adherence to medical advice. On the other hand, engaging the patient and asking about her understanding of the diagnosis and treatment plan is a way to make the patient a partner in the process. At the end of each counseling session, whether it is a sick visit or maintenance, I ask the parent (patient) to relate how they would explain the diagnosis and treatment to a significant other not present, like a partner, spouse, or grandparent. I believe this is more patient-friendly than asking the patient or parent to explain or repeat back what you just said. I also ask if there is anything in the diagnosis and treatment plan that the patient doesn't agree with or feels they cannot do. As an example, prescribing a medication three times a day might be perplexing for the patient or parent, as the child may be dropped off for daycare at 6:45 AM and not picked up until 6:00 PM. The question might be how to get in three doses of the medication during the day. This is a realistic and great question, and my response is usually one dose before daycare, one on arriving home, and one at bedtime. Of course, some medications have to be specific hours apart (e.g., every six hours during waking hours), and therefore, finding an alternative is reasonable (e.g., giving one dose in the morning, determining if the daycare can give a dose at noon, and then giving the third dose upon arrival at home).

The lesson here is to use questions to activate patients in the counseling process and to try to assess if the patient has concerns or misunderstandings about anything you have said. This kind of communication promotes trust and allows the patient to take responsibility for understanding the content of the visit and being able to explain the essence of the visit to a significant other.

Tip 24: Don't Teach Defensive Medicine to Trainees in Order to Avoid Malpractice Suits

I don't believe in so-called defensive medicine and have never practiced that way. In my almost 50 years of practice seeing tens of thousands of patients, I have been fortunate to have never been sued despite caring for very ill and complex patients, some of whom had poor outcomes. There is so much technology in medicine today, and it is so easy to depend on that to diagnose and treat patients. I believe in the tradition in getting trainees to focus on obtaining a great history and doing a thorough physical exam before entertaining any laboratory tests or imaging studies. On rounds, I often hear trainees rushing through the history and physical, and then moving right into the lab studies without hearing anything about their differential diagnosis and what they feel are the most likely diagnoses. How does one know what laboratory or imaging studies to order if the differential diagnosis is not clear? When one orders a complete blood count, based on the most likely diagnosis, what would one expect the count to show? There shouldn't be many surprises from laboratory study results when we deal with patients.

In addition, hearing histories and physical exams presented, I always identify gaps that need to be discussed with the trainee. Some of these gaps are key to making certain the initial assessment is correct. I teach that doing a complete history and physical is the essence of great medicine; nothing replaces that skill. Knowing how to observe appropriately before touching the patient, how to percuss a chest and abdomen correctly, how to convey information to patients, how to make certain one has established the patient's main concern and why that concerns her, and how to learn all the nuances of doing a great history and physical are the keys to practicing quality medicine, not defensive medicine. Never once have I ordered a test because of concerns of malpractice. That leads in nicely to the next story.

I had examined a school-aged patient who had had an episode of falling and hitting his head. It was not a high-velocity fall, he was never unconscious, he had no memory loss, and he remained coherent from the accident to the hospital visit. I took an exhaustive history; did a thorough physical exam, with attention to the neurologic and funduscopic exam; and made my assessment of head trauma without evidence of a concussion. The mother asked for a CT scan of the head, and I told her I did not feel any further studies would enhance the diagnosis or treatment I had made. She was adamant that she wanted a CT scan for her child, and I again assured her that I was treating her child no differently than I would have treated someone in my own family. The impasse persisted, and I asked if she wanted to speak with a patient representative, and she did. I explained the situation to the patient representative and told her that if the mother wanted to seek care elsewhere (likely an adult-oriented emergency room), she would be certain to get what she wanted. This does not represent the power differential that seems to exist between doctor and patient but an attempt to assure the patient that you have done all the necessary exams and tests to confirm the diagnosis. Once that reaches no resolution, there are patient advocates in most hospitals who can intervene and be a more neutral listener to the patient's story. The bottom line is you have to do what you feel is medically indicated based on the information you obtain and not bow to patient wishes that may be more emotionally laden.

Lessons learned: Over time and with practice, CEs can fine-tune their history and physical skills by having someone observe them interacting with a patient. With feedback on these observations, you should feel more comfortable with these skills and less dependent on technology. Some of this improvement might require revisiting Bates' or other textbooks on physical diagnosis, and certainly putting your knowledge into practice is critical. Also, reflecting on the process physicians experience every day is important for your growth and how you teach these skills. For example, after doing a thorough history and performing a complete physical exam, you should be thinking about the most likely diagnoses and the pathophysiology in the patient's illness. Once that is clear in your mind (i.e., is this inflammation, cancer, vascular, etc?), you then think about what laboratory tests and/or imaging studies might be useful and cost-effective in confirming what you were thinking. Again, based on your thoughts, you should be able to predict some of the lab results, like the hemoglobin (based on your exam of the nailbeds and mucous membranes), the white blood cell count (high if one suspects infection and normal if it's genetic), and urine studies (if the review of systems does not suggest genitourinary involvement).

Based on my life experiences, I urge you not to practice defensive medicine or teach those habits to trainees. It increases the costs of medicine and uses technology inappropriately. I hear from friends way too frequently about how their physicians misuse antibiotics or do excessive testing (my perceptions) on what seem to be straightforward problems. This inappropriate use of testing places greater burden on our lab and imaging departments and, unfortunately, does not equate to a better return on investment in most instances. Delving more into testing should happen when the diagnosis is unclear and the patient is not getting better. Most often, time has a way of healing, and having the patient check back by phone after 24 to 48 hours is important.

Tip 25: When the Diagnosis Is not Clear, I Never Tell the Patient that I Do not Know What the Problem Is

A story to illustrate this point: A practitioner once told me that early in his career, he was seeing a young preschool patient with fever, brought in by his grandparents. He took a complete history and did a thorough physical exam, not finding a source for the fever. The child did not appear severely ill despite his high temperature. When the grandparents asked him what the problem was, he answered, "I don't know." They responded, "Could you please send me to a physician who does know?" This story really sticks out in my mind because as we traverse important historical information and the physical exam, we are unconsciously, the more seasoned we are, eliminating some diagnoses and entertaining others. The child in this story had the classic diagnosis of fever of unknown origin, and most of these episodes resolve or culminate in benign diagnoses, like roseola. Occasionally, the patient does not get better over the next 48 hours, and then the practitioner has to entertain and pursue other diagnoses, like a urinary or occult bacterial infection. The fact is that doing a thorough history and physical exam on every patient helps to eliminate many possible diagnoses, and the physician can reply, "The diagnosis is not clear at this time, but I know that your child does not have anything considered severe or life-threatening. In the next 48 hours, we will have a better understanding of what is going on. I need to hear from you tomorrow or if your child gets sicker."

Lessons learned: There is a difference between telling parents or patients, "I don't know the diagnosis" and "the diagnosis at this point is not clear." In instances where the diagnosis has not yet manifested itself, physicians strive to make the patient comfortable and stress that keeping in touch is critical, especially if the patient is not improving or is getting worse. In my opinion, this approach does not interfere with the patient's trust and confidence in the doctor that has developed over time and mandates that the physician communicate clearly to the patient what he is thinking.

Tip 26: Assess Whether Patients Have not only Understood Your Instructions or Diagnosis but Are Able to Convey Them to a Significant Other, Spouse, or Relative with Whom They Are Living

I ask a number of questions at the closure of an interaction with a patient to make certain the patient or parent understands what I have said and can convey that to someone of importance to them. Those questions are the following:

1. Is there anything I have said that you don't understand or don't agree with?
2. Is there anything I have suggested that you are unwilling or unable to do?
3. When a spouse or significant other asks you what the doctor said, what will you tell them?
4. How do you pay for your prescriptions?

All these questions relate to the patient's understanding of what you have conveyed and perhaps identify some hurdles in not being able or willing to adhere to the medical advice. This approach also avoids the somewhat pejorative question, in my opinion, of "Could you repeat back to me what I just told you?" Lastly, knowing if the patient has medical insurance to cover the cost of any drugs prescribed is important. If that is not the case, I have always contacted social work to see if there is a way for them to help in this situation. As caregivers, we are remiss in not knowing more about drug prices, especially over-the-counter drugs, which are extremely expensive for populations that are not afflu-ent. Knowing what the patient can afford and what the price of the drug might be is helpful in problem-solving this issue.

ADMINISTRATIVE RESPONSIBILITIES AND LEADERSHIP

Tip 27: When Someone in Leadership Schedules a Meeting with You, Make Certain You Know the Agenda

Here are two stories that illustrate this point. The first story transpired at the mid-point in my career when the chief medical officer at Children's Hospital announced he was leaving the institution. The chair of the department called me into his office to discuss how to cover the responsibilities of that position until a new person was hired. I told him that I considered myself a team player and would be happy to assume some of the responsibilities in concert with other faculty. I left feeling like I had offered the chair my services in a couple of areas. A week later, I was informed that a meeting was to be scheduled with the chief executive officer. Again, I did not know the agenda, but I postulated in a conversation with my wife that he was going to offer me the job of chief medical officer, which I did not want. When I entered his office the following week, both he and the chair of the department were present. As expected, the chief executive officer told me he felt I was the most qualified person to take this position, and my emotional response that I had already volunteered to subsume some responsibilities went for naught. No job description or even salary was mentioned at that meeting, and it became a fait accompli. I was relieved of patient care duties, was not able to pay much attention to my role as head of the Office of Medical Education, and had to put my educational scholarship on hold. Six months later, the chief operating officer offered me the job permanently at $50,000 more salary. Using the George H. W. Bush famous phrase, "Read my lips," I replied that I was not interested.

Story 2 began when a new chair of pediatrics was hired at our hospital. I was called by his administrative assistant when I was seeing patients, and she asked if I could immediately meet with the incoming chair. I responded that it was not an optimal time to leave my scheduled patients. She said it was urgent, and so I finished with the patient I was seeing and attended the meeting. In essence, I was offered an important leadership position in education under the chair's new administration.

In doing due diligence, I asked to see my job description (of course, after telling the incoming chair I was flattered by the offer). He stated that there was no job description at that time, but he needed to know my answer immediately so he could announce it to the faculty the next day. I reluctantly agreed to the position without knowing my specific roles, responsibilities, and expectations. Basically, I was not able to reflect on my personal mission statement and decide if the new chair's vision of education was in sync with mine.

In fact, over time, I discovered that the new chair and I had conflicting ideas on how education should evolve in the institution, which created friction in carrying out my duties. For example, he asked why my strategic plan did not address the financing of resident education, way beyond the scope of an institutional medical education strategic plan. When we both realized the tension regarding our visions, I suggested we have a six-month moratorium, and after that time, I would decide if staying vice chair of education was in my best interests and that of the institution. In the end, I resigned from that position and felt like a load was removed from my shoulders. I went back to doing what I loved: working on patient care, running the Office of Medical Education, and engaging in educational scholarship, eliminating the administrative obligations and conflicts I had with the chair. Following that decision, I had an amiable relationship with the chair over time.

Lessons learned: I believe it is great advice to junior faculty to be vigilant about knowing the agenda when they are invited to a meeting. In both of my stories, unexpected demands were placed on me that made it difficult to respond adequately in the moment. Although you want to be known as a team player in the department, it is critical to ensure you have referred back to your mission statement in answering questions about important career options and have time to do so, perhaps discussing the decision with critical stakeholders. Of course, one can make exceptions when the circumstances are unusual. However, it is best to be prepared when, as a junior faculty member, you are not negotiating from a position of power. Thus, a word to the wise based on experience.

Tip 28: Network with Like-Minded Faculty Nationally by Getting Involved in Your Specialty Society's Annual Meetings and/or the Association of American Medical Colleges Annual or Regional Meetings

Through national organizations, faculty can network with others who have similar positions in their home institutions and who have some of the same challenges. There is common ground in several major areas: tips on how to recruit faculty to participate in focused faculty development programs, such as giving feedback, facilitating orientation of new learners, dealing with problem learners, writing balanced summative evaluations, and other issues focused on improving teaching and learning in the institution; ideas on how to encourage leadership to support the educational mission; suggestions on how to overcome barriers to conduct educational scholarship; discussion of models to achieve the Accreditation Council for Graduate Medical Education competencies and milestones for trainees; and ways to ensure recognition for educational efforts through promotion on the CE track. Networking has led to many instances of developing innovative programs, collaborative educational scholarship, and lifelong friends.

Tip 29: Think about Getting Some Leadership Training by Reading Books/Articles or Taking Workshops that Address Leadership in Medicine, an Often-Overlooked Area

It is indeed a sad commentary that medical school and residency training have provided little to no background in leadership skills. Basic issues on time management, leading a meeting, problem-solving an area that needs to be addressed, and group decision-making are just a few topics that enable us to be better at what we do. Dr. Carole Bland, a wonderful medical educator, wrote a book in the Springer series on how to be a successful faculty member. She included leadership skills in that book, which is still in print. By learning these skills, you can not only enhance your career but use them in administrative and clinical activities. In my personal experience, learning some of these skills allowed me to be a more effective administrator and teach them to others through faculty development workshops. Our colleagues in other disciplines, such as the business, health science, and educational schools in our academic community, can offer their expertise in areas that are not commonplace in medicine. In fact, I list in the annotated bibliography at the end of the primer a book from the Harvard Business School that focuses on case-based teaching, an example of how fields outside of medicine can make significant contributions to who we are as CEs.

In terms of enhancing your career, as you get more experience with time, your mission statement can change, and you can consider new adventures, such as residency program director or other leadership positions. Having experience with leadership skills in your portfolio can be an asset in your credentials for a move upward in the system.

Lessons learned: Leadership training is now available at many national meetings and likely within one's university setting. These skills are an asset for any level of CE but become more valuable as one aspires to assume more responsibility in that area, like chairing a committee in the department or medical school. As one seeks leadership opportunities nationally, having such a skill set can be helpful in carrying out the goals of the committee or task force that one chairs. There are also books that focus on leadership, which I have used to complement my knowledge and skills, such as *The Creative Techniques Handbook*.

Tip 30: Incorporating Group Decision-Making Techniques into Your Knowledge and Skill Sets Can Be Valuable

In my educational and leadership experiences, I have discovered the importance of learning and applying decision-making techniques that promote effective closure to issues the group is considering. Some of these include brainstorming, paired weighting, action learning, and the Delphi technique. I have used many of these techniques in committee work and, on occasion, in the educational domain. As CEs progress to leadership positions, it is comforting to know that they have tools to assist decision-making.

Short story: When invited to a university (not a medical school) to conduct faculty development sessions as part of the week devoted to education, I was asked to facilitate a workshop for a medical subspecialty group who had a problem that involved the teaching of resident physicians. I heard their dilemma and decided to use action learning, a technique developed by Dr. Marquardt at George Washington University Graduate School of Education and Human Development (see annotated bibliography later). The model depends on formulating a specific question for the organization that involves an unresolved problem, needs to be addressed in a timely manner, and is important to the stakeholders in that organization. Those participating in the process ($N = \sim 8$) need to be diverse and represent a wide range of people in the organization. The highlight of the process is that everyone gets many opportunities to pose questions around the problem, with the only discussion on each question related to clarification issues. This process continues until participants cannot generate any further questions. Then the group decides how to investigate those questions where answers are not readily known and reconvenes to problem-solve the issue once information is obtained. The limiting factor with the workshop is that it in itself is the beginning of the process, and all answers are not known at the conclusion of the workshop. Most of us look for a quick fix when we are addressing problems.

After I left, the division never informed me if the process was continued. Five years later, at a national meeting, one of the leaders of that division approached me to tell me they had used the model and solved the problem.

Lessons learned: The feedback from my action learning workshop reinforces the importance of using known techniques to approach difficult problems. Having these kinds of tools can be an asset as one accepts leadership responsibilities (dean positions, committee chairs, task forces, etc.). Knowing it is likely that many CEs at the mid-career stage will be chairing committees and task forces, it is important to have leadership skills that enhance that work.

Tip 31: As Mid-Level and Senior CEs, It Is Important that You Delegate to More Junior CEs and Senior Residents the Responsibility for Different Aspects of the Mission (Especially Around Teaching and Patient Care), Even Though It May Be Easier for You to Do the Work

I have often wanted to just do it instead of delegating responsibility to others. I know, based on my work ethic and organizing skills, that I get things done in an efficient and effective manner versus waiting for long periods of time for others to do the same work. However, this handoff process has to happen if we are to assure that the next generation continues the work that needs to be done in an excellent manner. Holding back is hard to do and is a learned phenomenon, especially for CEs who are committed and passionate about their work. It's so easy to just jump in and tell the team what the answer is to a particular problem. Just remember what level you are as a CE, and that should help in determining how you interact in a group regarding patient care or teaching. I have stated previously that having learners commit to the diagnosis is a key to assessing where they are regarding this patient's problems. Just keep in mind that learning is not about what *you* know; it's about what more junior people know and how they apply that to patient care and education.

PERSONAL LIFE

Tip 32: Always Keep in Mind Your Personal Life-Work Balance

It is so easy to get caught up in the responsibilities we all accept as part of our jobs in academic medicine that at times, we can devote inadequate time to our personal lives. Again, your mission statement can help define who you are as a CE. Sometimes, we have to say no to offers we find very attractive but at the expense of our own personal well-being and our relationships with family, friends, significant others or spouses, and children. Although I do not have a specific story to use as an example here, I was heavily involved in educational scholarship. My mantra was working smarter and not harder by including others in my work, which reduced the time needed on my part. Of course, I devoted time to educational scholarship on weekends and at nights, but I was also there for my children and wife. I coached sports, attended our children's life events that occurred throughout their education, and spent significant time with my wife, doing things together we both enjoy (gardening, theater, concerts, and travel). As we get older, we all have some regrets in not spending enough time with family. I somehow found the balance that I am addressing in this tip.

Lessons learned: Keeping your professional and personal life balance is so important, especially if you choose to have children. I can tell you as a senior citizen that the older one gets, the faster time seems to fly. As your children traverse critical periods of their development, you often have *one* opportunity to be there for them. I am suggesting that you keep your priorities in tow and make certain colleagues assume their share of night or weekend call, scholarship activities, and teaching, allowing you to honor commitments to family. It's sad when, on reflection, one shows remorse for not being present for important family milestones and joyous events that have occurred over the years.

Personally speaking, I worked very hard starting and overseeing an Office of Medical Education (one of the first in pediatrics in the country providing services across the continuum of education), seeing patients, doing educational scholarship, and teaching. My home activities centered mostly on creating new curricula, doing my nonfunded educational scholarship, and handling administrative responsibilities within the Office of Medical Education. I also made a conscious effort to consult part-time to supplement my salary at the medical center, and that work was done on nights and weekends. I believe my work ethic was a model in that I arrived at work at 7:00 AM and was seldom home before 6:00 PM, participated in night and weekend calls, yet managed my time well, spending time with family and addressing my professional responsibilities. I made time to coach baseball, soccer, and basketball, even though basketball was the only sport that I really knew well. It gave me an opportunity to be with our son, as he was interested in sports. In those days, even though our daughter was athletic, she refused to play organized sports and deprived me of coaching her. So, I was busy with personal and professional activities, but I managed to develop a balance that was rewarding in so many ways. I never missed a major milestone or even less important activities of my children, and I can say the same for my grandchildren. No regrets.

Tip 33: Benchmark Your Position When You Have Concerns about Pay Equality

Depending on pay raises, which often accompany promotions or are cost-of-living adjustments, you may at some point question whether your pay is equitable to that of others in the institution and nationally. The Association of American Medical Colleges has published salaries yearly for different specialties and at specific academic levels, differentiating women from men. Women are definitely compensated at lower salaries than men for each of the academic levels and lag behind in academic positions compared with men. As I have stated earlier, while it is best to negotiate a starting salary as high as possible, revisiting these numbers with time related to equity of pay and to what is comparable nationally can be enlightening. Determining what others in the same geographic area and academic positions receive in salary is a great starting point.

Here's a short story to illustrate this point. At the mid-level of my career, I had accomplished a lot for the institution, having started a community rotation for medical students and residents, and established an Office of Medical Education at Children's. I started to question how the institution was compensating me based on my track record. When I approached the chair of pediatrics, he suggested that I benchmark what I was doing compared with similar faculty nationally. I forewarned him that I knew of no other pediatricians doing the same depth and breadth of medical education, research-wise, teaching, or administratively. I contacted two peers, both younger than me, who were involved in education but not at the same level as the office I founded, which provided expertise across the continuum of education. Both confided confidentially that they were receiving salaries greater than $50,000, more than mine. When I reported this disparity back to the chair, he committed to raising my salary. Of course, when you decide to address this issue with leadership, you have to have confidence in what you have accomplished and how you have contributed to the department and medical school. It is possible that the chair will not be willing to discuss your salary and contributions in terms of a raise. So, you have to have flexibility to perhaps seek other employment if you find yourself stuck with no viable options for increased salary and/or moving upward in the division or department.

Lessons learned: Regarding your salary and how you are viewed within the department, if you don't ask, you won't know. On the other hand, you have to be comfortable and confident in your position within the division or institution to go down this path. At the time, I was nationally known and well published, and was ready, although not totally committed, to move on if there was no action on this issue. Procuring a pay raise addresses that issue, but more substantially, it also confirms the institution's valuing you and what you do.

Tip 34: Be Sure to Thank Those Who Have Mentored You, Briefly or in an Ongoing Fashion

Thank your mentors, and thank the outstanding teachers in your life, both in your role as a trainee and beyond. When faculty in your home and outside institutions have written supportive letters for you for promotion, let them know you appreciate it and send them a note when you hear about the committee's decision. The number of times I wrote supporting letters and never heard back about the promotion decision is too numerable to count. Need I say more?

Very often, fellow academicians have made a major impact on our careers, and due to many excuses, we don't seem to take the time to thank them for their contributions. Calling or emailing these influencers about promotions, awards, publications, and other achievements in your career is a way of saying thank you. In academia, we all seem to be on the fast track with all our responsibilities and long work weeks, and may not pause to think about how others have influenced us. Whereas many inherent factors influence where we are career-wise, others in our sphere have played a major role and contributed to our success story. These could include family members, significant others, teachers along the way, and colleagues.

Short story: Two people who were very important mentors to me both died prematurely and without warning. Each mentored me at different times early in my career: one conducted faculty development workshops at George Washington University on lecturing skills and became a coauthor on early research I conducted on learning styles and career choices, and the other pushed me to accept a leadership position in the Northeast Group on Educational Affairs after failing the first time around. I thanked each prospectively for being there for me, but as time passed, I lost track of both until I heard about their deaths.

Short story about just-in-time mentoring: During my mid-career time as a CE, I was invited to the University of California at San Francisco as a visiting professor in medical education. When I arrived at the center, David Irby, PhD, renowned medical educator and professor at UCSF, met me, and we immediately drove to Fresno, an affiliated hospital some four hours away, where I was to do a workshop on the problem learner. We arrived late, and the next morning, I prepared for the workshop, not immediately realizing that Dr. Irby was going to observe me facilitating the workshop. Talking about being nervous—performing before one of the top medical educational gurus in the world! I don't remember much about the details of the workshop, but once I finished facilitating, Dr. Irby provided me with just-in-time feedback and mentoring about my performance. Interestingly, the UCSF medical center had asked me to facilitate the same workshop on the main campus the following day, which I did, incorporating Dr. Irby's suggestions. He again observed my performance, noting if I had incorporated the feedback he had given me the day before. My vivid recollection of the experience suggested that this truly was a critical incident teaching moment. I was so grateful that he invested so much time in my performance, and I thanked him profusely.

I have another short story about my senior English teacher in high school (we're talking circa 1958) who also taught a drama class. We read so many wonderful plays and books, and I remember her as a benevolent task master with clear expectations. She really impacted how I appreciate literature and helped to establish a wonderful foundation for me by making all those works available. Sadly, I never thanked her and only recalled all those exciting and stimulating teaching moments when I saw her obituary in the local newspaper.

Lessons learned: We, as faculty, are never too expert or experienced to receive mentoring and feedback from peers. In the classic article in the *New Yorker* some years ago, Dr. Atul Gawande described seeking coaching from a former retired department chair in surgery to improve his performance, despite his many years of experience. In my case at UCSF, whereas I hadn't expected this in-the-moment mentoring to occur, I welcomed it nervously and am so happy in retrospect that it happened. So, a suggestion to mid-level CEs is to ask your peers who have similar interests to watch you perform a history and physical, facilitate a workshop or formal teaching session, conduct rounds, or chair a meeting. Once this has occurred and you have incorporated behavior change, you can add this to your educator portfolio as documentation of ongoing professional growth. More senior faculty seldom, if ever, receive feedback on performance, which in itself is sad. One of the mantras of medicine is the work ethic of continuing professional education, meaning that ongoing growth is critical to our professional identity and search for excellence. Feedback should be welcomed any time in our careers, and thanking those who provide this for us is being a consummate professional.

Finally, there was so much more I could have said to my mentors who died prematurely, and I missed that opportunity. Don't let that happen to you. Reach out to your mentors periodically. As you progress up the academic ladder, your life doesn't get less busy, and it can be easy to forget issues like this. Sending off an email or text can suffice, with actual conversations or in-person meetings not always imminent.

Tip 35: Take Joy in What You Do, Bringing Meaning to Your Professional Life

I cannot imagine my career bringing me more joy or sense of accomplishment than what I experienced over these 46 years as a CE. I have felt this way prospectively and upon reflecting on my career once retired. I would suggest that if you find that you are not getting meaning and joy out of your career, it's time to step back and reflect on your mission statement and how you see yourself going forward. I never looked at my job as work because I loved doing what I did every day. Don't get me wrong;

there were many struggles and clashes along the way, many of which were uncomfortable and far from joyous. However, and my spouse can back me up, I adhered to what I thought was right and did not give in to those who didn't value education and what I was doing. Sticking to principles allowed me to have such a wonderful career, balancing patient care, teaching, educational scholarship, and advocacy (to which I devoted much less attention because of all my other responsibilities).

A story illustrates my joy in working and sticking to my path. The first time I was eligible for promotion to full professor on the non-tenure track was in the mid-1980s, during my mid-career as a CE. Up until that point, I had published 45 original articles and numerous abstracts and had attained national recognition through my educational scholarship and educational activities. The chair of surgery, internationally known, contacted me after I was told that my promotion to professor was rejected and wanted to meet with me. He related that members of the appointment, promotion, and tenure committee were not familiar with some of the educational journals in which I published (e.g., *Journal of Medical Education*, *Medical Education*, and *Medical Teacher*), and he advised that I align myself with colleagues in subspecialties and conduct research in those areas. I remember replying that my passion was medical education, that it was not up to me to educate committee members about educational journals, and that I was going down a path from which I would not veer, promotion or not. Those who wrote letters of support for me were astounded that my promotion was turned down. It was gratifying to know that colleagues appreciated my work and were advocates for my promotion. That is what happens when one becomes involved nationally. Turns out that I did get promoted to full professor two years later, again during my mid-career tenure.

Lessons learned: Whereas I never considered what I did as work, there were times that tried my soul, especially with those to whom I reported. People have different visions of medical education, and one of the downsides of my career was trying to convince those in leadership positions of the virtues of education in an evidence-based way. I saw myself as a change agent after my meeting with Dr. George Miller, and that was one of the enjoyable parts of what I did (i.e., encouraging colleagues and trainees to adopt educational principles through covert infiltration). I saw it happen at my own institution and when I was a visiting professor. Whenever I was invited as a visiting professor—and I was fortunate enough to have visited two-thirds of US and some Canadian medical schools—I seized that opportunity to proselytize and present education as an integral and important part of one's academic specialty.

Those achievements of being promoted, being recognized for my efforts, and networking with so many valued colleagues were essential pieces of making my career so satisfying. Once those feelings stop, it is time to reevaluate and determine next steps. That might mean seeking employment elsewhere or changing directions in your current job, like seeking other opportunities, such as obtaining a master's in medical education or business administration. I was at an institution for 44 years, and the path that I followed is not a likely one with today's faculty. Lateral and upward moves to other institutions always remain a viable option for faculty who need a change of venue.

Ten Helpful Books

In this final section, I would like to recommend ten books that were helpful to me as a clinician educator (CE). (This is a sampling; there were many more.) Some can be read from cover to cover and others just as a reference. Each contributed to my knowledge about education, leadership, and educational scholarship.

1. **Knowles MS, Holton EF, Swanson RA.** *The Adult Learner: The Definitive Classic in Adult Education and Human Resource Development.* **5th ed. Gulf Publishing Co; 1998.**

   This is a classic work on the underpinnings of learning and teaching, and Knowles' theory of andragogy. Early in my career, Knowles' writings helped me understand the role of the teacher in interacting with learners, developing an approach on what to teach. Focusing on the learner was not the framework for most of us in my generation; rather, the mantra was "How do I improve my teaching?" Whereas Knowles never studied his model, his work is universally taught in undergraduate and graduate education. This is not a book that one would necessarily read from cover to cover, but it can be used as a frame of reference for different topics. As an example, the authors devote a chapter to the concept of learning contracts (see tips), an effective way to activate learners and stimulate their thinking on what they want to learn over a set period.

2. **Boyer EL.** *Scholarship Reconsidered. Priorities of the Professoriate.* **Jossey-Bass; 1990.**

   This booklet was my introduction to the concept of educational scholarship, as defined by Boyer's studies in his role as head of the Carnegie Foundation. Based on data he gathered on university faculty and their efforts regarding research, he

101

developed a model and defined educational scholarship as a way to broaden the definition of traditional research, identifying the following categories: (1) the scholarship of discovery, or what has been termed "research"; (2) the scholarship of application; (3) the scholarship of teaching, as opposed to teaching excellence; and (4) the scholarship of integration. In formulating educational scholarship in my career, I consciously refer back to this framework and have found it very useful. Many of my studies fit nicely into Boyer's classification of scholarship. His premature death led to the following book by Glassick, which addresses how one evaluates educational scholarship.

3. **Glassick CE, Huber MT, Maeroff GI.** *Scholarship Assessed: Evaluation of the Professorate. An Ernest Boyer Project of The Carnegie Foundation for the Advancement of Teaching.* **Jossey-Bass; 1997.**

   The authors define the characteristics of excellence in scholarship through adequate preparation, appropriate methods, significant results, effective presentation, and reflective technique. The importance of this and Boyer's work frames educational scholarship in a very positive and measurable way, and represents the basis for how CEs can document their educational activities and delineate their educational scholarship.

4. **Knowles M.** *Self-Directed Learning: A Guide for Teachers and Learners.* **Follett; 1975.**

   This 135-page handbook addresses self-directed learning as part of Knowles' andragogy theory. He addresses objectives, the learning contract, the development of self-directed learners, the learning climate, and the teacher's role as facilitator.

5. **Foley RP, Smilansky J.** *Teaching Techniques: A Handbook for Health Professionals.* **McGraw-Hill; 1980.**

   Richard Foley was a mentor to me, and I have used his book extensively in my teaching and workshops. I believe it is still available through Amazon. The book covers important areas, like lecturing, teaching a skill, principles of learning, how to use questions in one's teaching, and other important topics. I have used this handbook extensively in formulating workshops and teaching and learning innovations, and as a guide for understanding specific areas of medical education. It is geared to the clinician and provides basics about each subject matter in a concise way. It is 40 years old and not outdated.

6. **Schon DA.** *Educating the Reflective Practitioner.* **Jossey-Bass; 1987.**

This book is one of the most powerful influences on my career. Understanding how reflection, as a humanistic habit, can affect your behavior is the essence of how change can occur. Reflection-in-action and reflection-on-action for teaching and patient care represent forms of self-assessment in the moment and after the interaction. The concept of reflection-for-action came later as a way to project how one's performance can be even better in the future with a similar scenario.

7. **Barnes LB, Christensen CR, Hansen AJ.** *Teaching the Case Method.* **3rd ed. Harvard Business School Press; 1994.**

I have mentioned how other disciplines can inform us as medical educators, and this book is a classic example of that principle. The Harvard Business School is well known for the case-based method of teaching, and this book captures the essence of how the model works. Chapters are titled "Thinking in Education" by the famous educator John Dewey, "Teachers Must Also Learn", "Premises and Practices of Discussion Teaching", and "Why Teach?" This book is a sleeper, and I would guess most CEs have never heard of it. The book points out that teaching and learning are based on universal principles that cross disciplines. Delving into cases and then discussions is really the heart of the book. In medicine, we have exactly the same model, with the patients as the center of our teaching and care. All patients are unique and come to the healthcare system with different sets of symptoms, personal characteristics, support systems, and preferences for how they like to interact with healthcare professionals. The point is that cases allow for contextual learning, and the Harvard Business School learned that long ago. I found the book at icobooks.com.

8. **Marquardt M.** *Leading with Questions.* **Jossey-Bass; 2005.**

This is one of my favorite books around the leadership theme. Marquardt, a fellow George Washington University faculty member in the Graduate School of Education and Human Development, is the guru of action learning, a wonderful technique in solving problems he has applied with Fortune 500 companies. I have learned the technique and presented it in workshops at a number of academic health centers, teaching faculty how to approach solving difficult problems. A faculty member at a university where I spoke saw me five years afterward at a national meeting and told me the technique worked. I wish there were more feedback like that. Without getting into the details of the model, suffice it to say that it focuses on a problem in an academic health center that is important to many, needing expedient attention and problem-solving, and requiring stakeholders (N = 8) from a variety of backgrounds across the center to participate in the model. The questioning process by participants is the backbone of the model and the most important issue before any problem-solving or efforts to seek solutions are attempted.

9. **Tiberius RG. *Small Group Teaching: A Trouble-Shooting Guide*. The Ontario Institute for Studies in Education; 1990.**

   I had heard Richard Tiberius, an experienced professional educator from Toronto (more recently, professor emeritus, the University of Miami Miller School of Medicine), speak in the 1990s, and that is where I heard about his book on group teaching. It is very detailed regarding what to expect in a small group session and how the facilitator can think about responding. Obviously, teaching in this setting is very different from teaching one-on-one. Those CEs who teach in inpatient units with a team, such as on the general medicine wards, need to know how small groups function and how faculty need to be mindful of group dynamics, engaging all team members, refining questioning skills, and addressing the milestones and competencies. It would be an understatement to recognize the multitasking necessary for faculty in this setting. The book seems more focused on classroom teaching, but the educational and interactional principles apply anywhere.

10. **Whitman N, Schwenk TL. *The Physician as Teacher*. 2nd ed. Whitman Associates; 1997.**

    This concise handbook was first published in the late 1980s and was written by a professional educator and the chair of family practice in a Midwest academic health center who is very invested in medical education. It addresses important issues in a one-stop shop book that includes the responsibilities of the physician, communication with patients, teaching rounds and morning report, and teaching in the ambulatory and inpatient units. This is a great reference and source for specific areas of teaching and learning.

Epilogue

Having spent my entire career as a CE and making medical education the focus of my professional being was so rewarding for me and provided a niche that allowed me to develop a professional identity. This is not a path one takes alone, but this is a path that evolves into collaborations and so many relationships within and outside your field. Some of these colleagues become close friends. In fact, I have been fortunate to have made longtime friends that go back more than 40 years.

Although I have some regrets about my performance in specific workshops, patient encounters, or teaching interactions (reflection-on-action), I have no regrets about a wonderful career and my personal life as a husband, father, and grandfather. I made mistakes along the way that might have been avoided had I had more experience and wisdom at the time. But the fact that I had so many stories to tell that were learning experiences was the major vector that morphed into this primer. I hope that my stories, tips, and lessons learned are helpful to CEs at different stages of their careers. Stories highlighting experiences can be powerful in making connections with others. Readers can resonate with stories "That sounds familiar; I have been in that situation." Most importantly, translating what you have learned from the primer into action and creating change as you search for excellence are the real essence of my story.

I wish you the best of luck in your career as a CE and hope you find the same joy and meaning that I did. Stay true to your mission statement over time, treat colleagues and trainees with respect, be there for your family, and be creative as you pursue your goals. As Robin Williams' character said in the film *Dead Poets Society*, "carpe diem."

Index

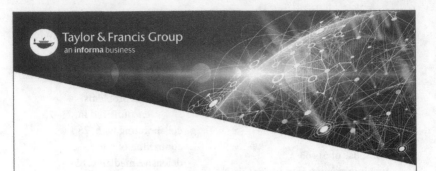

Printed in the United States
by Baker & Taylor Publisher Services

Printed in the United States
by Baker & Taylor Publisher Services